Practical Pharmaceutical Calculations
SECOND EDITION

MICHAEL BONNER
Lecturer in Pharmaceutics
School of Pharmacy
University of Bradford

and

DAVID WRIGHT
Senior Lecturer in Pharmacy Practice
School of Chemical Sciences and Pharmacy
University of East Anglia

Radcliffe Publishing
Oxford • New York

Radcliffe Publishing Ltd
18 Marcham Road
Abingdon
Oxon OX14 1AA
United Kingdom

www.radcliffe-oxford.com
Electronic catalogue and worldwide online ordering facility.

First edition 1999 (published by LibraPharm Ltd)

British Library Cataloguing in Publication Data

A catalogue record for this book is available from the British Library.

ISBN-13: 978 184619 251 7

Typeset by Pindar New Zealand (Egan Reid), Auckland, New Zealand
Printed and bound by TJI Digital, Padstow, Cornwall, UK

Practical Pharmaceutical Calculations

Contents

Preface

We are happy to introduce the second edition of *Practical Pharmaceutical Calculations* which, since its first publication in 1999, has sold in excess of 20,000 copies. After consultation with students, pharmacists and university teachers our second edition is altered to begin with a new chapter on fundamental arithmetical and mathematical operations needed for successful progression through each of the subsequent chapters. As before, self-assessment calculations are provided at the end of each chapter along with their fully worked solutions.

This edition also seeks to develop both the student's mental arithmetic and mathematics. The authors hope that the reader will carry out all the questions contained in each chapter as far as possible without the aid of an electronic calculator. We wish to remove dependence of students on calculators in order that they develop a better 'concept of magnitude' or, in other words, that they can readily perceive if their answer to each problem is a credible one. The experience of the authors is that many students will accept without question answers given by a calculator without considering if they are realistic.

Note that in order to provide calculations to be performed by students on pen and paper alone, we have approximated some physical constants, e.g. atomic weight of potassium, displacement values of medicaments in suppositories, and so our colleagues with an understandable desire for scientific accuracy are offered apologies in advance.

Michael Bonner
David Wright
January 2008

About the authors

Dr Michael Bonner has been a lecturer in Pharmaceutics at the University of Bradford since 1997, where he teaches various aspects of the discipline, including extemporaneous dispensing. His research interests include breaching the skin's barrier to drug penetration and formulation of strategies to maximise bioavailability by this route. He has been a registered pharmacist since 1991.

Dr David Wright undertook his PhD and formative years as a lecturer in pharmacy practice at the School of Pharmacy in Bradford. More recently he has been responsible for the undergraduate professional curriculum at the University of East Anglia, the first new school of pharmacy to graduate pharmacy students in the UK for over 30 years.

1

Fundamentals of arithmetic and algebra

Develop a concept of magnitude: is the answer a credible one?

As you work through this book, one of the skills you should develop is an ability to estimate a credible answer. This is, of course, not only useful in the context of this book but also in everyday life. Consider the following situation:

> In a clothes shop you buy five items priced at: £17, £22, £18, £23 and £19. How much do you estimate you will pay?
>
> Is it: £25, £50, £100, £200 or £400?

> If you look at the cost of each of the five items you will see that each costs approximately £20, so the total cost should be roughly £20 × 5 = £100. If you can readily estimate the cost, then you can detect if you are ever over- or under-charged. If you can't readily estimate the cost, you could quickly become poorer!

Let us now consider a more pharmaceutical example:

> A patient weighing 61 kilograms needs a drug dosage of 20 milligrams per kilogram of body weight. Estimate how much total drug the patient should receive.
>
> Is it: 200, 400, 600, 800 or 1200 milligrams?
>
> The patient weighs approximately 60 kilograms so requires approximately 20 mg × 60. (If you can't readily multiply

3

by 60, multiply by 10 and then by 6.) If the patient weighed 10 kilograms he would need 20 mg × 10 = 200 milligrams.

A 60-kilogram patient therefore requires 200 mg × 6 = 1200 milligrams. So, a credible answer is 1200 mg.

A credible estimate is not a wild guess, but rather a sensible answer based on the information presented to you. In this instance the true answer was of course 1260 milligrams, but you are much less likely to cause harm to the patient with a reasonable estimate within 5% of the correct answer than one with an error of 50%, 100% or 900%.

You may think that you are unlikely to give an answer which is incorrect by 900% but a 10-times overdose (or underdose) is just that. Such an error is more likely to occur when a student relies heavily upon a calculator, and then accepts the calculator's answer without question. Therefore, we urge you to practise the examples throughout this book *without* the use of a calculator and, when you believe you have answered a question, ask yourself, 'Is this a credible answer?'

The rest of this chapter is devoted to a brief overview of basic arithmetic and algebra necessary for successful completion of subsequent chapters. If there is any part of this first chapter that you have difficulty with, we suggest you refer to the very useful textbook *The Sciences Good Study Guide.*[1]

Fractions

Fractions express proportions of whole items. For example, you have a disc drive with 400 GB storage capacity and have 100 GB of files stored on it. The fraction of the storage space used on the disc can be written as

$$\frac{100}{400}$$

The number above the line is known as the numerator, while the number below the line is known as the denominator. In this example you can consider 100 to be the 'proportion' of the 'whole' 400. If the numerator is larger than the denominator the fraction is called a 'vulgar fraction', e.g.

$$\frac{18}{4}$$

Equivalent fractions

If you consider the previous example of $\frac{100}{400}$, note that if you multiply (or divide) the numerator and denominator by the same number the fraction retains the same value.

So $\frac{100}{400} = \frac{200}{800}$ (as we have multiplied top and bottom by 2), which is also equivalent to $\frac{1}{4}$ as we have now divided both numerator and denominator by 200.

Note that throughout this book you may find rather 'ugly' fractions such as $\frac{25}{0.01}$. It has often been this author's experience that when a student is asked to evaluate such a fraction, they shudder. To evaluate these fractions, the principle is the same as before: multiply top and bottom of the fraction until manageable whole numbers are obtained. Multiplication by 10 is generally most useful.

So, $\frac{25}{0.01} = \frac{250}{0.1} = \frac{2500}{1} = 2500$ (we have multiplied top and bottom by 10 each time).

Simplifying fractions: 'cancelling down'

It is generally easier to work with fractions when the numerator and denominator are as low as possible. This is achieved by repeatedly dividing numerator and denominator by the same number to obtain smaller whole numbers until this is no longer possible. It is usually easiest to attempt to divide top and bottom by small numbers such as 2, 3, 4, 5 or 10.

Example 1.1   Simplify as far as possible $\frac{24}{96}$

Solution steps

1   Look at numerator and denominator and check if both are readily divisible.

2   Repeat step 1 until the fraction is in its simplest form.

As both 24 and 96 are even numbers, both are divisible by 2.

So, $\frac{24}{96} = \frac{12}{48} = \frac{6}{24} = \frac{3}{12}$

Now, both numerator and denominator are divisible by 3 so $\frac{3}{12} = \frac{1}{4}$

The fraction is now in its simplest form.

Percentages

In a similar manner to fractions, percentages represent proportions of whole items, e.g. if 90% of students passed an examination it would mean that 90 out of every 100 students who sat the examination had passed it. Note that the 'whole' does not have to be 100 items. If 200 students had taken the examination and 180 had passed it, that would also represent 90%.

Decimals

Decimals are a way of representing (normally) numbers which are not whole numbers. The use of a decimal point separates the whole number from the parts of the decimal which are not whole, for example 1.25 grams of a drug means we have 1 gram of it, plus two-tenths of a gram, plus five hundredths of a gram. Note that if the *only number* before the decimal point is zero, we are considering a quantity which is less than one, e.g. 0.25 grams of a drug is less than one gram and represents the two tenths and five hundredths of a gram as before.

Conversion between fractions and decimals

Any decimal (or any whole number for that matter) can be converted to a fraction by simply putting the decimal over a denominator of 1.

Example 1.2   Convert 0.25 into a fraction in its simplest form

Solution steps
1 Write 0.25 as a decimal.
2 Make an equivalent fraction by multiplying top and bottom by 10 until decimal point is removed.
3 Simplify the fraction by division.

Hence, 0.25 can be written as $\frac{0.25}{1}$. Now evaluate this as before:

$\frac{0.25}{1} = \frac{25}{10} = \frac{25}{100}$ (multiply the top and bottom by 10).

You should be able to see that this can be readily simplified:

$\frac{25}{100} = \frac{5}{20} = \frac{1}{4}$ (divide the top and bottom by 5).

To convert a fraction into a decimal simply divide the numerator by the denominator. It may be necessary to write the numerator as a decimal with one or more zeroes after the decimal point in order to carry out the division.

Example 1.3   Express $\frac{2}{5}$ as a decimal

Solution steps
1 Try to divide the numerator directly by the denominator. If the numerator is smaller than the denominator, write the numerator as a decimal with one or more zeroes after the decimal point in order to carry out the division.

So write 2.0, divide this by 5 and you should obtain 0.4. You could have written 2.00 by five and obtained an answer of 0.40, which is equivalent to 0.4. In some cases you will never obtain an answer that ends in zero and you could be writing the answer for an infinite time, e.g. if you express 1/3 as a decimal the answer is 0.33333 . . .

recurring. In this book, most answers will be given to two decimal places (number of digits after the decimal point), unless the division process can be completed with no remainders, e.g. if you express 1/8 as a decimal you will obtain exactly 0.125.

Conversion between fractions and percentages

To convert from a fraction to a percentage is very straightforward. Simply multiply the numerator by 100 and evaluate the fraction as before and express this with a % sign.

Example 1.4 Express $\frac{4}{5}$ as a percentage

Solution steps
1 Multiply numerator by 100.
2 Evaluate fraction as a number (or decimal).
3 Place a % sign after the value.

So, $\frac{4}{5}$ becomes $\frac{400}{5}$ = 80, hence this is 80%.

Note that a percentage can have a decimal point in it, e.g. $\frac{305}{1000}$ = 3.05%.

Similarly, converting from a percentage to a fraction is straightforward. Divide the number by 100, then express the fraction in its simplest terms.

Example 1.5 Express 55% as a fraction

Solution steps
1 Divide numerator by 100.
2 Simplify the fraction.

So 55% becomes $\frac{55}{100}$; if we simplify this becomes $\frac{11}{20}$ which cannot be simplified any further.

Conversion between decimals and percentages

To convert decimals to percentages, the quickest approach is to multiply the decimal by 100 and place a % sign after the answer.

Example 1.6   Express 0.6 as a percentage

Solution steps
1   Multiply by 100.
2   Add a % sign.

0.6 multiplied by 100 gives 60%.

Simply reverse the steps for conversion from percentages to decimals.

Example 1.7   Express 12% as a fraction

Solution step
1   Divide by 100.

So, $12\% = \frac{12}{100} = 0.12$

Here we could have simplified the fraction to $\frac{3}{25}$, but division by 100 is more straightforward than division by 25.

Elementary algebra

Algebra is a way of representing numbers through lettered symbols, e.g. a, b, c, x, y. The letters can then be used to represent relationships between the quantities through equations. Some of the simplest rules for handling algebraic expressions are given below.

$a + b = b + a$

$a \times b = b \times a$ (You may see these frequently written in algebra as $ab = ba$)

Note: $a–b \neq b–a$

$$\frac{a}{b} \neq \frac{b}{a}$$

So, addition and multiplication are both reversible operations (also called commutative) but subtraction and division *are not.*

$a^0 = 1$

$a^1 = a$

$a^2 = a \times a$

$a^3 = a \times a \times a$

or $a^3 = a^2 \times a^1$

The general rule is: $a^x \times a^y = a^{(x+y)}$

Conversely, the equation can be written thus:

$$\frac{a^x}{a^y} = a^{(x-y)}$$

Therefore:

$$\frac{a^3}{a^2} = a^{(3-2)} = a^1 \text{ or } a$$

$$a^{\frac{1}{2}} = \sqrt{a}$$

Manipulation of equations

An equation represents a relationship between quantities. Consider the following:

$$concentration = \frac{mass}{volume} \text{ OR abbreviate to } C = \frac{M}{V}$$

Frequently we may have to rearrange the equation to find an unknown quantity. In this case we have to make something else the *subject of the equation.* The key rule when rearranging equations is to do exactly the same process, e.g. an addition, subtraction, multiplication or division, to *both* sides of the equation (on either side of the equals sign).

Example 1.8 In the equation above, make *M* the subject of the equation

Solution steps
1 Decide what needs to be done to make *M* the subject. Carry out any process to make *M* stand alone on one side of the equals sign.
2 As M is being divided by *V* currently, multiply both sides by *V* to rearrange the equation.

So, $C = \dfrac{M}{V}$ therefore $M = CV$

Example 1.9 Make *u* the subject of the equation $s = ut + \frac{1}{2}at^2$

Solution steps
1 Decide what needs to be done to make *u* the subject. Carry out any process to make *u* stand alone on one side of the equals sign.
2 Subtract both sides by $\frac{1}{2}at^2$
3 Divide both sides by *t*

So, if $s = ut + \frac{1}{2}at^2$ then $s - \dfrac{at^2}{2} = ut$ so $u = \dfrac{s - \frac{at^2}{2}}{t} = \dfrac{s}{t} - \dfrac{at^2}{2t}$

so $u = \dfrac{s}{t} - \dfrac{at}{2}$

SELF-ASSESSMENT

Now try the self-assessment questions to ensure you have understood this chapter.

Questions

1 Give a reasonable estimate of how much white soft paraffin is in 1010 grams of an ointment if you know that 30% of the ointment comprises white soft paraffin.

2 A tube of ointment contains 48 grams of product. Estimate how many grams of ointment would be in 50 tubes.

3 125 grams of an ointment contain 25 grams of zinc oxide. Express the amount of zinc oxide as the simplest possible fraction and as a percentage.

4 Express 21 out of 105 as a decimal.

5 What is 22% as a decimal?

6 Express $\frac{18}{4}$ as a number with a decimal point.

7 Evaluate $\frac{0.12}{0.3}$

8 Express $\frac{2}{18}$ as a percentage (to three decimal places).

9 Make n the subject of the equation $PV = nRT$

10 Make c the subject of the equation $x = \frac{b^2 + 4ac}{2a}$

Reference

1 Northedge A, Lane A, Peasgood A, *et al. The Sciences Good Study Guide.* Buckingham: Open University Worldwide; 1997.

2

Units of measurement

By the end of this chapter, you should be able to:
- give the units of mass, volume and drug amount commonly used in pharmacy
- convert between larger and smaller units of mass, volume and drug amount.

The metric system

In the UK, the metric system is now most commonly used for the expression of quantities in pharmacy. For a particular quantity a base unit exists: the gram is the base unit of mass, the litre is the base unit of volume and the mole is the base unit for drug amount. Prefixes are used to indicate quantities greater or less than the base unit. Table 2.1 lists the prefixes most commonly used in pharmacy, and gives an example of each.

TABLE 2.1 Prefixes used in the metric system

Prefix	Denoting	Example
kilo	One thousand times greater than the base unit	kilogram
milli	One thousand times less than the base unit	millilitre
micro	One million times less than the base unit	micromole

The units of mass

The most commonly used units of mass are listed in Table 2.2.

TABLE 2.2 Units of mass

Unit	Abbreviated to	Equivalent to
1 kilogram	kg	1000 grams
1 gram	g	1000 milligrams
1 milligram	mg	1000 micrograms
1 microgram	µg or mcg	

Masses greater or less than these amounts are rarely used in pharmacy. To convert from smaller units to larger ones (e.g. milligrams to grams, grams to kilograms) we need to divide by 1000. Conversely, to convert from larger units into smaller ones (e.g. kilograms to grams, grams to milligrams) we must multiply by 1000 (*see* Figure 2.1).

Example 2.1   Add 0.00250 kg, 1750 mg, 2.50 g and 750,000 mcg
(express your answer in grams)

Solution steps
1   Convert each of the quantities to grams.
2   Add the converted quantities together.

0.00250 kg = (0.00250 × 1000) grams	= 2.50 grams
1750 mg = (1750 ÷ 1000) grams	= 1.75 grams
2.50 grams	= 2.50 grams
750,000 micrograms = (750,000 ÷ 1,000,000) grams	= 0.75 grams
Total mass	= 7.50 grams

Answer: 7.50 grams

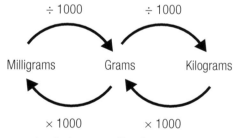

FIGURE 2.1 Conversion between units of mass

The units of volume

The base unit of volume is the litre (L). Table 2.3 gives the units of volume commonly used in pharmacy.

TABLE 2.3 Units of volume used in pharmacy

Unit	Abbreviated to	Equivalent to
1 litre	L	1000 millilitres
1 millilitre	mL	1000 microlitres

To convert volumes from litres into millilitres, we must multiply by 1000 and to convert volumes from millilitres into litres, we must divide by 1000 (*see* Figure 2.2).

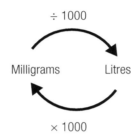

FIGURE 2.2 Converting between units of volume

Example 2.2 Add 3 L, 1150 mL and 0.75 L. Give the total volume in mL

Solution steps
1   Convert each of the quantities to millilitres.
2   Add the converted quantities together.

3 L = (3 × 1000) mL	= 3000 mL
1150 mL	= 1150 mL
0.75 L = (0.75 × 1000) mL	= 750 mL
Total volume	= 4900 mL

Answer: 4900 mL

Example 2.3 A patient is prescribed 10 mL of a mixture to be taken four times a day. How much of the mixture (in litres) is required to give the patient 30 days' supply?

Solution steps
1   Calculate how much the patient takes each day.
2   Calculate how much the patient then needs for 30 days.
3   Convert this figure from mL to L.

Each day the patient takes 10 mL × 4 = 40 mL

For 30 days the patient needs 40 mL × 30 = 1200 mL

1200 mL is equal to (1200 ÷ 1000) litres = 1.2 L

Answer: 1.2 litres

Units of drug amount

The base unit for an amount of drug is the mole. One mole is the amount of substance containing 6.02×10^{23} of its component formula units (e.g. atoms, molecules or ions). The number of moles of a drug may easily be expressed as a mass since a mole of a drug weighs, in grams, the same as the relative molecular mass (RMM) of the substance. Thus, for example, 1 mole of potassium chloride (RMM = 74.5) weighs 74.5 grams. Table 2.4 shows the units of drug amount commonly used in pharmacy.

TABLE 2.4 Units of drug amount

Unit	Abbreviated to	Equivalent to
mole	mol	1000 millimoles
millimole	mmol	1000 micromoles

Figure 2.3 shows the conversion between moles and millimoles, and their conversion into units of mass.

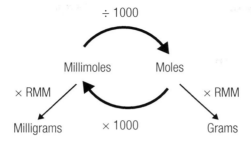

FIGURE 2.3 Converting between units of drug amount

Example 2.4   How many millimoles of potassium chloride (assume RMM = 75) are present in 150 grams of the substance?

Solution steps
1   Calculate the number of moles of the drug.
2   Convert this into millimoles.

75 grams is the weight of 1 mole of potassium chloride

1 gram is the weight of 1 ÷ 75 moles of potassium chloride

150 grams is the weight of 150 ÷ 75 moles of potassium chloride
= 2 moles

2 moles = (2 × 1000) millimoles = 2000 millimoles

Answer: 2000 millimoles

SELF-ASSESSMENT

Now try the self-assessment questions to ensure you have understood this chapter.

Questions

1 Add 7 kg, 75 g and 750,000 mcg. Give your answer in grams.

2 Add 0.04 L, 20 mL and 200 µL. Give your answer in mL.

3 A doctor prescribes 250 mg of minocycline to be taken four times a day for 20 days. Calculate the total weight of minocycline taken by the patient.

4 A capsule contains the following ingredients. Calculate, in grams, the amount of each ingredient required to manufacture 10,000 capsules:

Chlorpheniramine maleate   4 mg
Phenylpropanolamine hydrochloride   50 mg

5 A transdermal patch contains 8 mg of oestradiol. How many grams of oestradiol are required to make 50,000 patches?

6 An inhaler delivers 50 micrograms of salmeterol in each inhalation, and contains 200 metered inhalations. How many milligrams of salmeterol are present in the inhaler?

7 A patient is prescribed 15 mL of a mixture to be taken twice daily for 14 days. How much of the mixture should be supplied?

8 Sodium bicarbonate capsules each contain 600 mg of the compound. If a patient takes seven of these in a day, how many mmol of sodium bicarbonate has the patient taken? (RMM of sodium bicarbonate = 84).

9 An intravenous infusion contains 30 mmol of sodium chloride. What is the mass of sodium chloride (in grams) contained in the infusion? (RMM of sodium chloride = 60).

10 An effervescent tablet for oral rehydration contains 120 mg of sodium chloride and 150 mg of potassium chloride. How many mmol of *chloride* are contained in one tablet? (Take RMM of sodium chloride, NaCl, = 60, RMM of potassium chloride, KCl = 75).

3

Understanding concentrations

Expressions of concentration

The vast majority of the pharmaceutical preparations used in the UK contain an active ingredient (drug) dissolved or dispersed in a solvent or diluent. Various expressions may be used to define the concentration of a drug in a preparation and a knowledge of these is essential in the practice of pharmacy. Additionally, understanding expressions of concentration is also important when examining clinical laboratory test results, as biochemical results may be given in a variety of ways. In this chapter, we will consider four different ways of expressing concentrations:

- quantity per volume
- percentage concentrations
- parts
- ratios.

Quantity per volume

Quantity per volume expressions are used to give the concentration of drugs in solution and also for clinical laboratory test results. A quantity per volume expression gives the amount or weight of drug (in terms of moles or grams, respectively) in a volume of solution. For example, a 9 g/L solution of sodium chloride means that 9 g of sodium chloride are dissolved in 1 litre of solution. A 1 mmol/L solution of sodium chloride contains 1 mmol (equivalent to 0.058 g) of the compound dissolved in 1 litre of solution.

Example 3.1   What weight of sodium bicarbonate (in grams) is required to make 200 mL of a 6 g/L solution?

Solution steps

1 Look at the concentration expression and work out how much is contained in 1 mL of solution.
2 Calculate how much is required to make 200 mL of solution.

6 g/L means that 6 g of sodium bicarbonate must be dissolved in 1 litre (1000 mL) of solution.

So, 6 ÷ 1000 g of sodium bicarbonate must be dissolved in 1 mL of solution.

So, (6 ÷ 1000) × 200 g of sodium bicarbonate must be dissolved in 200 mL of solution.

Answer: = 1.2 grams

Example 3.2   A patient has a serum potassium level of 4 mmol/L. a) How many millimoles of potassium are present in a 20 mL sample of the patient's serum? b) How many milligrams of potassium are present in this sample? (RMM of potassium = 40)

Solution step a)

1 Look at the concentration expression and calculate how many millimoles are present in 1 mL of serum.
2 Calculate how many millimoles are present in 20 mL of serum.

4 mmol/L means that 4 mmol of potassium are present in 1 L of serum.

So, 4 ÷ 1000 mmol of potassium are present in 1 mL of serum.

Therefore, (4 × 20) ÷ 1000 mmol of potassium are present in 20 mL of serum.

80 ÷ 1000 mmol = 0.08 mmol.

Answer: 0.08 millimoles

Solution step b)
Convert the number of mmol to mg by multiplying by the RMM (*see* Chapter 2).

1 mmol of potassium weighs 40 mg.

0.08 mmol of potassium weigh 0.08 × 40 mg = 3.2 mg.

0.08 mmol of potassium are present in 20 mL of serum.

Answer: 3.2 mg of potassium are present in 20 mL of serum

Percentage concentrations

Percentages may be used to express drug concentration in both liquid and solid dosage forms. A percentage concentration denotes the number of parts of a drug (either as grams or millilitres) in 100 parts of the dosage form. Three different percentage concentrations are commonly used, and their use depends on the nature of the product.

% w/v

Percentage weight in volume, used to express the weight of a solid in 100 mL of a liquid product. For example, a 1% w/v solution of sodium chloride in water denotes that 1 g of sodium chloride is contained in 100 mL of solution. To make this solution, 1 g of sodium chloride would be dissolved in a small volume of water, and the solution made up to 100 mL with water.

% w/w

Percentage weight in weight, used to express the weight of a solid, or occasionally a liquid, in 100 g of a solid product. For example, a 1% w/w hydrocortisone ointment denotes that 1 g of hydrocortisone is contained in 100 g of the final ointment. To make this product 1 g of hydrocortisone would be mixed with a small weight of the ointment base and then the product would be made up to 100 g with further ointment base.

% v/v

Percentage volume in volume, used to express the volume of a liquid in 100 mL of a liquid product. For example, an emulsion containing 50% v/v liquid paraffin denotes that 50 mL of liquid paraffin are contained in 100 mL of the final emulsion.

Example 3.3   A mouthwash contains 0.1% w/v chlorhexidine gluconate. How much chlorhexidine gluconate in grams is contained in 250 mL of the mouthwash?

Solution steps
1   Look at the concentration expression and determine how much drug (in grams) is contained in 1 mL of the product.
2   Calculate how much drug would therefore be contained in 250 mL of the product.

0.1% w/v denotes that 100 mL of the mouthwash contains 0.1g of chlorhexidine gluconate.

So, 1 mL of the mouthwash contains (0.1 ÷ 100) g of chlorhexidine gluconate.

Therefore, 250 mL of the mouthwash contains (0.1 ÷ 100) × 250 g of chlorhexidine gluconate = 0.25 g.

Answer: 0.25 grams

Example 3.4   What weight of miconazole is required to make 40 g of a cream containing 2% w/w of the drug?

Solution steps
1   Look at the concentration expression and determine how much drug is contained in 1 g of the product.
2   Calculate how much drug would therefore be contained in 40 g of the product.

2% w/w denotes that 100 g of the cream must contain 2 g of miconazole.

So, 1 g of the cream must contain 2 ÷ 100 g of miconazole.

Therefore, 40 g of the cream must contain (2 ÷ 100) × 40 g of miconazole.

Answer: 0.8 grams

Example 3.5 How much arachis oil is required to make 300 mL of an emulsion containing 30% v/v of arachis oil?

Solution steps
1 Look at the concentration expression and determine how much arachis oil is contained in 1 mL of the product.
2 Calculate how much arachis oil would therefore be contained in 300 mL of the product.

30% v/v denotes that 100 mL of the emulsion contains 30 mL of arachis oil.

So, 1 mL of the emulsion contains 30 ÷ 100 mL of arachis oil.

Therefore, 300 mL of the emulsion contains (30 ÷ 100) × 300 mL of arachis oil = 90 mL.

Answer: 90 millilitres

Ratio concentrations

A ratio concentration is most commonly used to express the concentration of very dilute solutions. It expresses the number of parts (usually millilitres) of a solvent within which one part of the drug (usually grams) is dissolved or dispersed. Thus, a 1:5000 solution of a drug indicates that 1 g of the drug is dissolved in 5000 mL (5 L) of solution.

Example 3.6   How many milligrams of adrenaline are contained in 10 mL of a 1:10,000 solution of the drug?

Solution steps

1   Convert the ratio to a quantity per volume expression.
2   Calculate how much adrenaline is present in 1 mL of the solution.
3   Calculate how much adrenaline is present in 10 mL of solution.

A 1:10,000 solution denotes that 1 g of adrenaline is dissolved in 10,000 mL of the solution.

So, 1 mL of the solution will contain 1 ÷ 10,000 g of adrenaline.

Therefore, 10 mL of the solution will contain (1 ÷ 10,000) × 10 g of adrenaline = 0.001 g = 1 mg.

Answer: 1 milligram

Parts as expressions of concentration

This method of expressing concentrations is similar to ratio expressions except that the convention is to replace the ratio symbol with the word 'in'. Thus, a 1:1000 solution becomes a 1 in 1000, but the meaning is unchanged, i.e. 1 g of a drug dissolved in 1000 mL of a solution.

Example 3.7   A 10 mL ampoule of a 1 in 200,000 solution of bupivacaine hydrochloride is administered to a patient. How many milligrams of bupivacaine hydrochloride does the patient receive?

Solution steps

1   Convert the parts expression to a quantity per volume expression.
2   Calculate how much bupivacaine hydrochloride is present in 1 mL of the solution.
3   Calculate how much bupivacaine hydrochloride is present in 10 mL of solution.

A 1 in 200,000 solution denotes that 1 g of bupivacaine hydrochloride is dissolved in 200,000 mL of the solution.

So, 1 mL of the solution will contain $(1 \div 200,000)$ g of bupivacaine hydrochloride.

Therefore, 10 mL of the solution will contain $(1 \div 200,000) \times 10$ g of bupivacaine hydrochloride = 0.00005 g = 0.05 mg.

Answer: 0.05 milligrams

Converting between expressions of concentration

It is frequently necessary to convert between the various expressions of concentration. In order to do this, you should ensure that you understand what is meant by each of the expressions of concentration described previously.

Example 3.8   A solution contains 10 mg of drug in 5 mL of solution. Express this as a ratio concentration.

Solution steps

1   Determine what concentration expression is required.
2   As a ratio concentration is required, determine what volume of solution would contain 1 g of drug.
3   Express this as a ratio.

10 mg of the drug is contained in 5 mL of the solution.

So, 1 mg of the drug is contained in $5 \div 10$ mL of the solution.

Therefore, 1 g of the drug is contained in $(5 \times 1000) \div 10$ mL of the solution = $5000 \div 10$ mL = 500 mL.

Answer: 1:500

SELF-ASSESSMENT

Now try the self-assessment questions to ensure you have understood this chapter.

Questions

1 A patient is prescribed a suspension containing 2 mg/mL of a drug. The directions are for the patient to take 10 mL of the suspension three times a day for one week. How many milligrams of the drug will the patient receive in the week?

2 A patient dissolves two tablets, each containing 300 mg of aspirin, in 120 mL of water. What is the aspirin concentration (% w/v) of the solution?

3 How many grams of an antibiotic are required to prepare 50 mL of a 0.25% w/v solution of the antibiotic?

4 A liniment contains 5% v/v methyl salicylate. How much methyl salicylate is required to make 600 mL of the liniment?

5 How much hydrocortisone is present in 120 g of a cream containing 0.5% w/w hydrocortisone?

6 Sodium chloride infusion 0.9% w/v is used widely for electrolyte replacement. Express this concentration of sodium chloride in mmol/L. (Take RMM of sodium chloride = 60)

7 What volume of a 1:20,000 solution of adrenaline would contain 50 mg of the drug?

8 What is the % w/v concentration of a 1000 mmol/L solution of sodium bicarbonate? (RMM of sodium bicarbonate = 84)

9 A patient uses 200 mL of a 1:8000 solution of an antiseptic, daily, for 10 days. How many grams of the antiseptic have been used?

10 You are provided with a powdered drug which contains 10% w/w moisture. What weight of the powder do you need to make 5 L of an aqueous solution with a concentration of 4% w/v of the *anhydrous* drug?

4

Formulae for extemporaneous dispensing

By the end of this chapter you should be able to:
- use a reference source formula to calculate quantities of each ingredient required to make a given amount of a pharmaceutical product
- correctly interpret formulae where ingredient quantities are listed as parts or percentages.

Reference source formulae

When a pharmaceutical product is to be prepared extemporaneously, a reference formula is usually required. These formulae can be found in the pharmaceutical reference sources, such as the *British Pharmacopoeia* or the *Pharmaceutical Codex*. A reference formula lists the ingredients of the preparation and the quantities of each ingredient required to make a certain weight or volume of the preparation, depending on whether the preparation is a solid or a liquid. Frequently, the weight or volume of the preparation given in the reference formula will not be the same as that which must be prepared, in which case the quantities of each ingredient must be increased or reduced.

Example 4.1   You are asked to prepare 300 mL of Single Strength Chloroform Water. The formula is given below:

Concentrated Chloroform Water	25 mL
Purified water	to 1000 mL

Solution steps
1   As this is a liquid preparation, calculate how much of each component is required to make 1 mL of the product.
2   Calculate, therefore, how much is required to make 300 mL of the product.

Conc. Chloroform Water	25 mL	25 ÷ 1000 mL	(25 ÷ 1000) × 300 mL	7.5 mL
Purified water	to 1000 mL	to 1 mL	to 300 mL	to 300 mL

Note: we have effectively multiplied the Concentrated Chloroform Water quantity by 300/1000 or 0.3.

Example 4.2 You are required to prepare 5000 g Zinc Cream BP. The formula is given below:

Zinc oxide	320 g
Calcium hydroxide	0.45 g
Oleic acid	5 mL
Arachis oil	320 mL
Wool fat	80 g
Purified water to produce	1000 g

Solution steps

1   As this is a solid preparation, calculate how much of each component is required to make 1 g of the product.

2   Calculate therefore, how much is required to make 5000 g of the product.

Zinc oxide	320 g	320 ÷ 1000 g	(320 ÷ 1000) × 5000 g	1600 g
Calcium hydroxide	0.45 g	0.45 ÷ 1000 g	(0.45 ÷ 1000) × 5000 g	2.25 g
Oleic acid	5 mL	5 ÷ 1000 mL	(5 ÷ 1000) × 5000 mL	25 mL
Arachis oil	320 mL	320 ÷ 1000 mL	(320 ÷ 1000) × 5000 mL	1600 mL
Wool fat	80 g	80 ÷ 1000 g	(80 ÷ 1000) × 5000 g	400 g
Purified water	to 1000 g	to 1 g	to 5000 g	to 5000 g

Note: here in effect we multiplied each quantity required by 5.

In the above two examples, the final line of the reference formula indicates that the product is to be made up to a certain weight or volume. However, this may not always be the case. Consider the formula for Hydrous Ointment BP in Example 4.3. The total weight of the ingredients is 1000 g, so the quantities of each ingredient must be scaled up or down, based upon how much of the product is required.

Example 4.3   You are required to dispense 50 g of Hydrous Ointment BP. The formula is given below:

Wool alcohols ointment	500 g
Phenoxyethanol	10 g
Dried magnesium sulphate	5 g
Purified water	485 g

Solution steps
1   Add together the quantities of each ingredient.
2   Divide the quantity of each ingredient by this sum to find how much of each ingredient would be required to make 1 g of the product.
3   Calculate the amounts required for 50 g.

Total weight of the ingredients is 1000 g. Therefore:

Wool alcohols ointment	500 g	500 ÷ 1000 g	(500 ÷ 1000) × 50 g	25 g
Phenoxyethanol	10 g	10 ÷ 1000 g	(10 ÷ 1000) × 50 g	0.5 g
Dried magnesium sulphate	5 g	5 ÷ 1000 g	(5 ÷ 1000) × 50 g	0.25 g
Purified water	485 g	485 ÷ 1000 g	(485 ÷ 1000) × 50 g	24.25 g
Total weight	1000 g	1 g	50 g	50 g

Note: here we have effectively divided each quantity by 20.

Formulae in parts or percentages

Occasionally, the respective amounts of the ingredients are listed as either parts or percentages. This type of formula is usually written by a prescriber requesting 'special' ointments or creams.

Example 4.4   Prepare 30 g of the following ointment

Hydrocortisone ointment	25%
White soft paraffin	50%
Liquid paraffin	25%

Solution steps

1   Work out the quantities of each ingredient that would be required to make 100 g of the product – these will be the same as the percentages.
2   Calculate the amounts required for 30 g.

Hydrocortisone ointment	25%	25 g	$(25 \div 100) \times 30$ g	7.5 g
White soft paraffin	50%	50 g	$(50 \div 100) \times 30$ g	15 g
Liquid paraffin	25%	25 g	$(25 \div 100) \times 30$ g	7.5 g
Total weight		100 g	30 g	30 g

Example 4.5   Prepare 400 g of the following cream:

Betamethasone cream	1 part
Aqueous cream	3 parts

Solution steps

1   Sum the total number of parts.
2   Divide the number of parts of each ingredient by this sum to obtain a fraction.
3   Multiply this fraction by the required weight of the product to find the weight of each ingredient required.

Total number of parts = 4

Required weight of betamethasone cream $= \frac{1}{4} \times 400 = 100$ g

Required weight of aqueous cream $= \frac{3}{4} \times 400 = 300$ g

SELF-ASSESSMENT

Now try the self-assessment questions to ensure you have understood this chapter.

Questions

In each case, calculate the quantities of each component required to make the required amount of the preparation

1 Prepare 250 mL of Acid Gentian Mixture BP.

Acid Gentian Mixture BP
Concentrated compound gentian infusion	100 mL
Dilute hydrochloric acid	50 mL
Double strength chloroform water	500 mL
Water	to 1000 mL

2 Prepare 150 mL of Potassium Citrate Mixture BP.

Potassium Citrate Mixture BP
Potassium citrate	300 g
Citric acid monohydrate	50 g
Lemon spirit	5 mL
Quillaia tincture	10 mL
Syrup	250 mL
Double strength chloroform water	300 mL
Water	to 1000mL

3 Prepare 300 mL of Chloral Elixir Paediatric BP.

Chloral Elixir Paediatric BP
Chloral hydrate	200 mg
Water	0.1 mL
Blackcurrant syrup	1 mL
Syrup	to 5 mL

4   Prepare 200 mL of Paediatric Ferrous Sulphate Mixture BP.

Paediatric Ferrous Sulphate Mixture BP

Ferrous sulphate	60 mg
Ascorbic acid	10 mg
Orange syrup	0.5 mL
Double strength chloroform water	2.5 mL
Water	to 5 mL

5   Prepare 50 g of Coal Tar and Zinc Ointment BP.

Coal Tar and Zinc Ointment BP

Strong coal tar solution	100 g
Zinc oxide	300 g
Yellow soft paraffin	600 g

6   Prepare 600 g of Zinc and Salicylic acid paste BP.

Zinc and Salicylic acid paste BP

Zinc oxide	24%
Salicylic acid	2%
Starch	24%
White soft paraffin	50%

7   Prepare 20,000 mL of Magnesium Hydroxide Mixture BP.

Magnesium Hydroxide Mixture BP

Magnesium sulphate	47.5 g
Sodium hydroxide	15 g
Light magnesium oxide	52.5 g
Chloroform	2.5 mL
Water	to 1000 mL

8   Prepare 30 g of the following ointment:

Fluocinolone acetonide cream	10%
Aqueous cream	to 100%

9 Prepare 75 g of the following cream:

Betamethasone cream	1 part
Aqueous cream	4 parts

10 Prepare 80 g of the following ointment:

Dithranol ointment	1 part
White soft paraffin	to 4 parts

(Caution: Read the second line of the formula carefully.)

5

Dilution, mixing and incorporation

By the end of this chapter you should be able to:
- carry out calculations involving dilution of solutions and solid preparations
- carry out calculations involving mixing of solutions and solid preparations
- carry out calculations involving incorporation of medicaments into solid preparations.

Dilution of solutions

The dilution of solutions is one of the most frequently carried out calculations in pharmacy. A stock solution, or concentrate, must often be diluted to a particular strength for patient use. This type of calculation is particularly common for antiseptic and disinfectant preparations. In a dilution, the weight of the active ingredient will stay the same throughout; therefore, a simple formula for these calculations may be derived.

(*Note:* in the questions in this chapter we are assuming no contraction or expansion of volumes associated with the dilution processes.)

Mass of active before dilution = mass of active after dilution

However: Conc. of active = Mass of active ÷ Volume of solution

Thus: Mass of active = Conc. of active × Volume of solution

So: (Before dilution) Conc. of active (C_1) × Vol. of solution (V_1) = Conc. of active (C_2) × Vol. of solution (V_2) (after dilution)

Abbreviating: $C_1 \times V_1 = C_2 \times V_2$

For this equation to hold, both concentrations must be expressed in the same units and both volumes must also be expressed in the same units.

Example 5.1　How many millilitres of a 10% w/v solution of an antiseptic must be used to make 4 litres of a 0.25% w/v solution?

Solution steps

1　Fill in the appropriate values in the equation:
$$C_1 \times V_1 = C_2 \times V_2$$
2　Rearrange the equation to find the unknown (V_1).

$C_1 = 10\%$ w/v

$V_1 = ?$

$C_2 = 0.25\%$ w/v

$V_2 = 4$ litres

$10 \times V_1 = 0.25 \times 4$

Therefore, $V_1 = (0.25 \times 4) \div 10 = 0.1$ L $= 100$ mL

Answer:　100 millilitres

Example 5.2　How many millilitres of water must be ADDED to 250 mL of an 18% w/v stock solution of sodium chloride to prepare a 0.9% w/v sodium chloride solution?

Solution steps

1　Fill in the appropriate values in the equation
$$C_1 \times V_1 = C_2 \times V_2$$
2　Rearrange the equation to find the unknown (V_2).
3　As we need to find out how much water must be *added* to carry out the dilution, subtract 250 mL from V_2.

$C_1 = 18\%$ w/v

$V_1 = 250$ mL

$C_2 = 0.9\%$ w/v

$V_2 = ?$

$18 \times 250 = 0.9 \times V_2$

Therefore, $V_2 = (18 \times 250) \div 0.9 = 5000$ mL.

However, to carry out the dilution 5000 mL – 250 mL must be added = 4750 mL.

Answer: 4750 millilitres

Example 5.3   How many millilitres of a 1:5000 solution of phenylmercuric nitrate can be made from 250 mL of a 0.2% w/v solution of the compound?

Solution steps

1   Make the expressions of concentration similar.
2   Fill in the appropriate values in the equation
$C_1 \times V_1 = C_2 \times V_2$
3   Rearrange the equation to find the unknown (V_2).

A 1:5000 solution means that 1 g of the active is dissolved in 5000 mL.

So, $1 \div 5000$ g is dissolved in 1 mL.

Therefore, $(1 \div 5000) \times 100$ g is dissolved in 100 mL = 0.02 g in 100 mL = 0.02% w/v

$C_1 = 0.2$ % w/v

$V_1 = 250$ mL

$C_2 = 0.02$ % w/v

$V_2 = ?$

$0.2 \times 250 = 0.02 \times V_2$

Therefore, $V_2 = (0.2 \times 250) \div 0.02 = 2500$ mL.

Answer: 2500 millilitres

Dilution of solid preparations

Occasionally, a prescriber may request the dilution of active ingredients in a solid preparation. As the weight of active ingredient in the preparation will remain the same during the dilution, the following formula should be used.

(Before dilution) Conc. of active (% w/w) × Total mass of product = Conc. of active (% w/w) × Total mass of product (after dilution)

Abbreviating: $C_1 \times M_1 = C_2 \times M_2$

Example 5.4   You are supplied with 50 g of salicylic acid ointment 2% w/w. What weight of emulsifying ointment (diluent) should be added to reduce the concentration of salicylic acid to 0.5% w/w?

Solution steps
1   Fill in the appropriate values in the equation
    $C_1 \times M_1 = C_2 \times M_2$
2   Rearrange the equation to find the unknown (M_2).
3   As we need to find out how much emulsifying ointment must be added to carry out the dilution, subtract 50 g from M_2.

$C_1 = 2\%$ w/w

$M_1 = 50$ g

$C_2 = 0.5\%$ w/w

$M_2 = ?$

$2 \times 50 = 0.5 \times M_2$

Therefore, $M_2 = (2 \times 50) \div 0.5 = 200$ g.

However, to carry out the dilution 200 g – 50 g must be added = 150 g.

Answer: 150 grams

Mixing of solutions

If two or more solutions of the same active ingredient are mixed the final concentration of the ingredient may be calculated readily.

Example 5.5 What is the concentration of dextrose in a solution prepared by mixing 200 mL of 10% w/v dextrose, 50 mL of 20% w/v dextrose, and 100 mL of 5% w/v dextrose?

Solution steps

1 Calculate the weight of dextrose in each of the solutions to be mixed.
2 Calculate the total volume of the mixture produced.
3 From these, calculate the concentration of dextrose in the mixture.

10 % w/v dextrose will contain 10 g dextrose in 100 mL of solution.

Therefore, 1 mL of solution contains $10 \div 100$ g of dextrose.

So, 200 mL of solution contains $(10 \div 100) \times 200$ g of dextrose = 20 g of dextrose.

20% w/v dextrose will contain 20 g dextrose in 100 mL of solution.

Therefore, 1 mL of solution contains $20 \div 100$ g of dextrose.

So, 50 mL of solution contains $(20 \div 1000) \times 50$ g of dextrose = 10 g of dextrose.

5% w/v dextrose will contain 5 g of dextrose in 100 mL of solution.

So, 5 g of dextrose are present in this solution.

Total weight of dextrose = 20 g + 10 g + 5 g = 35 g.

Total volume of mixture = 200 mL + 50 mL + 100 mL = 350 mL.

The mixture contains 35 g of dextrose dissolved in 350 mL of solution.

Therefore, 1 mL of solution contains (35 ÷ 350) g of dextrose.

So, 100 mL of solution contains (35 ÷ 350) × 100g of dextrose = 10 g.

Answer: the mixture contains 10% w/w dextrose

A more common problem in pharmacy is one where a solution of a particular concentration is required, and it must be produced from a mixture of two other solutions.

Example 5.6   You are presented with a 500 mL infusion bag containing 5% w/v dextrose and a number of ampoules containing 10% w/v potassium chloride. A prescriber requests that sufficient potassium chloride is added to the infusion bag so that it will contain 0.2% w/v potassium chloride

*S*olution steps
1   Let the weight of potassium chloride required to be added = *x* grams.
2   Construct an equation where the final weight of potassium chloride in the bag divided by its final volume is equal to (0.2 ÷ 100).
3   Solve for *x*.
4   Calculate the volume of 10% w/v potassium chloride which must contain *x* grams.

The solution that must be produced is to contain 0.2 g potassium chloride in each 100 mL of solution. Irrespective of the final volume of the solution, this concentration must be obtained.

Let the weight of potassium chloride to be added to the bag = x grams.

The following equation can be constructed:

$$\frac{\text{Final weight of drug}}{\text{Final volume of solution}} = \frac{0.2}{100}$$

This is equivalent to:

$$\frac{\text{Initial weight of drug + added weight of drug}}{\text{Initial volume of solution + added volume of solution}} = \frac{0.2}{100}$$

Initial weight of drug in the bag = 0

Added weight of drug = x g

Initial volume of solution = 500 mL

Added volume of solution = $(100 \div 10)x$ mL or $10x$

Since, 10 g of potassium chloride are dissolved in 100 mL of the solution.

1 g of potassium chloride is dissolved in $100 \div 10$ mL of the solution.

Thus, x g of potassium chloride is dissolved in $(100 \div 10)x$ mL of the solution or $10x$ mL.

Substituting into the equation:

$$\frac{0 + x}{500 + 10x} = \frac{0.2}{100}$$

Cross multiplying:

$$0.2(500 + 10x) = 100(0 + x)$$

$$100 + 2x = 100x$$

Rearranging:

$98x = 100$

$x = 0.98$ g

0.98 g of potassium chloride are dissolved in $(100 \div 10) \times 0.98$ mL of the 10% w/v solution = 9.8 mL

Answer: 9.8 mL of the 10% w/v potassium chloride must be added to the infusion bag

Incorporation of medicaments into solid preparations

If we need to increase the concentration of an active ingredient in a cream or ointment by addition of pure extra ingredient, a calculation similar to Example 5.6 must be carried out. The next example will illustrate this point.

Example 5.7 What weight of coal tar extract must be added to 100 g of a cream containing 1% w/w coal tar extract to produce a cream containing 25% w/w coal tar extract?

Solution steps
1 Let the weight of coal tar extract to be added = x grams.
2 Construct an equation where the final weight of coal tar in the cream divided by the final weight of the cream is $25 \div 100$.
3 Solve for x.

The cream that must be produced is to contain 25 g of coal tar extract in each 100 g of cream. Irrespective of the final weight of the cream, this concentration must be obtained.

Let the weight of coal tar extract to be added = x grams.

The following equation can be constructed:

$$\frac{\text{Final weight of drug}}{\text{Final weight of cream}} = \frac{25}{100}$$

In this case, this is equivalent to:

$$\frac{\text{Initial weight of drug + added weight of drug}}{\text{Initial weight of cream + added weight of drug}} = \frac{25}{100}$$

Initial weight of drug = 1 g (since we have 100 g of a 1% w/w cream)

Added weight of drug = x g

Initial weight of cream = 100 g

$$\frac{1 + x}{100 + x} = \frac{25}{100} = \frac{1}{4}$$

Cross multiplying:

$4(1 + x) = 1(100 + x)$

$4 + 4x = 100 + x$

Rearranging:

$3x = 96$

$x = 32$ g

Answer: 32 grams

Example 5.8   What weight of coal tar extract must be added to 200 g of a cream containing 1% w/w coal tar extract to produce a cream containing 25% w/w coal tar extract?

Solution steps

1   Let the weight of coal tar extract to be added = x grams.
2   Construct an equation where the final weight of coal tar in the cream divided by the final weight of the cream is $25 \div 100$.
3   Solve for x.

The cream that must be produced is to contain 25 g of coal tar extract in each 100 g of cream. Irrespective of the final weight of the cream, this concentration must be obtained.

Let the weight of coal tar extract to be added = x grams

The following equation can be constructed:

$$\frac{\text{Final weight of drug}}{\text{Final weight of cream}} = \frac{25}{100}$$

In this case, this is equivalent to:

$$\frac{\text{Initial weight of drug} + \text{added weight of drug}}{\text{Initial weight of cream} + \text{added weight of drug}} = \frac{25}{100}$$

Initial weight of drug = 2 g (since we have 200 g of a 1% w/w cream)

Added weight of drug = x g

Initial weight of cream = 100 g

$$\frac{2 + x}{200 + x} = \frac{25}{100} = \frac{1}{4}$$

Cross multiplying:

$4(2 + x) = 1(200 + x)$

$8 + 4x = 200 + x$

Rearranging:

$3x = 192$

$x = 64$ g

Answer: 64 grams

SELF-ASSESSMENT

Now try the self-assessment questions to ensure you have understood this chapter.

Questions

1   How many millilitres of a 0.2% w/v solution of an antiseptic must be used to prepare 1 litre of a 1:5000 solution?

2   What volume of a 1:5000 solution of cetrimide can be made from 100 mL of a 4% solution of cetrimide?

3   A patient is directed to use 50 mL of a 1:10,000 solution of potassium permanganate solution twice a day for five days. You have in stock a 2% w/v solution of the compound. How much of the concentrate will you require to dispense the prescription?

4   How many millilitres of water must be *added* to 50 mL of 13% w/v aluminium acetate solution to prepare a 0.65% w/v solution?

5   How many grams of emulsifying ointment must be *added* to 200 g of 5% w/w calamine in emulsifying ointment, in order to reduce the calamine concentration to 2% w/w?

6   You have an infusion solution – volume 1 L – of 0.3% w/v potassium chloride and a number of ampoules containing 25% w/v dextrose. What volume of the 25% w/v solution of dextrose must be added to the infusion bag to produce a concentration of 5% w/v dextrose?

7   A prescriber requests that sufficient potassium chloride is added to 1000 mL of a 0.9% w/v sodium chloride infusion to give a final concentration of 40 mmol/L potassium. What volume of a 16% w/v potassium chloride solution should be added to the infusion? (Take RMM of potassium = 40)

8   A cream (weight 30 g) contains 0.1% w/w dithranol. What weight of dithranol powder should be added to increase the concentration to 1% w/w?

9 Salicylic acid ointment contains 2% w/w salicylic acid. What weight of salicylic acid powder should be added to 50 g of the ointment to produce a 10% w/w ointment?

10 A cream contains 10% w/w coal tar solution. What weight of coal tar solution should be incorporated into this cream to produce 30 g of cream containing 12% w/w coal tar solution?

6

Dose calculations

By the end of this chapter you should be able to:
- calculate doses for adult patients based on their actual and ideal body weight and their surface area
- calculate doses for paediatric patients based on their actual body weight and their surface area
- calculate infusion rates for intravenous drips and syringe pumps.

Dosage calculations

There are many drugs for which there are no standard doses, and for these drugs calculation of the dose required is dependent on a patient characteristic, such as body weight or surface area.

Example 6.1 What dose of salbutamol would you recommend for a 10 year old child, weight 30 kg, when the recommended dosage is 100 mcg/kg?

In this example the dose would be 30 kg × 100 mcg/kg = 3000 mcg = 3 mg

Example 6.2 What dose of vincristine is required for a 92 kg patient with a body surface area (BSA) of 2.0 m^2 and a recommended dosage of 1.4 mg/m^2?

In this example the dose would be 2.0 m^2 × 1.4 mg/m^2 = 2.8 mg

Table 6.1 summarises the most common dosage units based upon a patient's weight or surface area.

TABLE 6.1 Patient characteristics and corresponding dose units

Characteristics	Dose units	Abbreviated to
Weight	Grams per kilogram	g/kg
	Milligrams per kilogram	mg/kg
	Micrograms per kilogram	mcg/kg
	Units of drug per kilogram	U/kg
Body surface area	Grams per square metre of surface area	g/m^2
	Milligrams per square metre of surface area	mg/m^2
	Micrograms per square metre of surface area	mcg/m^2
	Units of drug per square metre of surface area	U/m^2

In Example 6.1 the patient's actual body weight (ABW) was used. In some instances it is more appropriate to use the patient's ideal body weight (IBW). Calculation of IBW is necessary for adult patients whose body weight is more than either 30% above or below the average adult weight of 70 kg (i.e. for obese or emaciated patients).

Where drugs are predominantly distributed in the lean tissues, e.g. drugs such as digoxin, the lower of either the ABW or IBW is used.

Calculation of ideal body weight

Ideal body weight (kg) is calculated from the patient's height (H, expressed in centimetres) using the following equation:

Males $IBW = (0.9 \times H) - 88$

Females $IBW = (0.9 \times H) - 92$

Estimation of body surface area

In Example 6.2 body surface area (BSA) was used and this is usually obtained from the patient's height and actual body weight. The patient's surface area can be determined from these two parameters by using one of two methods.

■ Nomograms for calculating BSA are provided in standard medical texts.[1] The same nomograms can be used for adults and children over one year old. Infants (less than one year old) generally have their own nomogram.

- One simple formula for estimating BSA,[2] provided below, is suitable for use in adults and children and is considered to be more accurate than the nomogram method. Height (H) in centimetres and weight (W) in kilograms are used to determine BSA (in square metres).

Surface area formula: $BSA = \sqrt{\dfrac{H \times W}{3600}}$

Example 6.3 The dosage of the chemotherapeutic agent cyclophosphamide can be expressed in mg/m² in some regimens and in mg/kg in other regimens. If the doses required are either 60 mg/kg or 800 mg/m² for a male adult patient who weighs 100 kg and measures 1.8 metres, give the three alternative doses to be administered based on ABW, IBW and BSA

Solution steps
1 Calculate the patient's IBW.
2 Calculate the patient's BSA.
3 Calculate the dose using ABW, IBW and BSA.

ABW = 100 kg

$BSA = \sqrt{\dfrac{H \times W}{3600}} = \sqrt{\dfrac{180 \times 100}{3600}} = \sqrt{5}$

IBW = $0.9H - 88 = (0.9 \times 180) - 88 = 74$ kg

BSA = 2.2 m²

Answers:

Dose based on ABW	= 100 × 60	= 6000 mg
Dose based on IBW	= 74 × 60	= 4440 mg
Dose based on BSA	= 2.2 × 800	= 1760 mg

Dose calculations for paediatrics

Paediatric doses are usually calculated on the basis of weight or surface area in a similar manner to the adult dose examples given in Table 6.1. As stated earlier, infants under one year old have a separate nomogram for the determination of surface area.

If however specific paediatric doses cannot be found, the percentage method of dose calculation is sometimes used. Table 6.2 shows the relationship between the average weight for a child's age and the percentage of the adult dose the child should receive.

TABLE 6.2 Percentage method for calculating doses[3]

Age	Mean weight for age (kg)	Percentage of adult dose
Newborn (full term)	3.5	12.5
2 months	4.5	15
4 months	6.5	20
1 year	10	25
3 years	15	33.3
7 years	23	50
10 years	30	60
12 years	39	75
14 years	50	80
16 years	58	90
Adult	68	100

Example 6.4   A three year old child of average weight is prescribed a drug for which there is no known paediatric dose. The adult dose of the drug is 600 mg daily. How much could you give the child using the percentage method of dose calculation (to the nearest milligram)?

Solution steps

1   Establish what percentage of the adult dose the child should receive.

2   Establish the normal adult dose.
3   Divide the quoted percentage by 100 and multiply by the adult dose.

A three year old of average weight should receive 33.3% of the adult dose.

The normal adult dose is 600 mg daily.

Dose for the child = (33.3 ÷ 100) × 600 = 199.8 or 200 mg daily.

Answer: 200 milligrams daily

Infusion rates

Some drugs, e.g. frusemide, phenytoin, potassium chloride and vancomycin, have maximum rates over which they can be infused. Infusion rates are usually limited as toxic effects may occur if the drugs are given too rapidly.

Doses for drugs such as dopamine and dobutamine used in acute situations are often expressed in quantity of drug to be delivered per kilogram of body weight per minute. It is important, therefore, to understand how to calculate infusion rates and give accurate advice about how these drugs should be delivered.

Example 6.5   A dose of 2 mcg/kg/minute of dopamine is required to be infused into an 80 kg patient over 100 minutes. What volume of dopamine 0.16% w/v infusion is required?

Solution steps
1   Calculate the total amount of dopamine required.
2   Identify the amount of dopamine in 100 mL of infusion.
3   Calculate the volume of infusion required to provide the total amount of dopamine required.

The patient requires 2 mcg/kg/min × 80 kg × 100 min = 16,000 mcg = 16 mg

In 100 mL of 0.16% w/v infusion there will be 0.16 g = 160 mg

Therefore, volume of infusion required = $\dfrac{16\,mg}{160\,mg} \times 100mL = 10mL$

Answer: 10 millilitres

Example 6.6 A dopamine infusion is set up for a 60 kg female, to deliver 2.5 mcg/kg/min. The syringe contains 200 mg dopamine in 50 mL normal saline. What should the infusion rate be in millilitres/hour?

Solution steps
1 Calculate the dose required in terms of mg/hour.
2 Establish the number of mg/mL in the dopamine infusion.
3 Divide the dose in mg/hour by the number of milligrams of dopamine in each millilitre of infusion to give the infusion rate in millilitres/hour required.

Dose required is 2.5 mcg/kg/min

= 2.5 mcg × 60 kg = 150 mcg/min

= 150 mcg × 60 min = 9000 mcg/h (or 9 mg/h)

Infusion contains 200 mg in 50 mL

= 200/50 mg in 1 mL = 4 mg/mL

Rate required = 9 mg/h ÷ 4 mg/mL = 2.25 mL/h

Answer: 2.25 millilitres/hour

Intravenous infusions which do not require as much accuracy in their delivery (e.g. routine fluid replacement or blood transfusion) are administered using standard giving sets and require calculation of drop rates. Drop volumes supplied by standard giving sets are given in Table 6.3.

TABLE 6.3 Drop volumes for standard giving sets

Adult	Paediatric	Blood
1 mL = 20 drops	1 mL = 60 drops	1 mL = 15 drops

Example 6.7 An adult giving set with fixed drop size and adjustable flow is being used to deliver 1.2 litres of normal saline over 10 hours. What should the drop rate be set at in drops/minute?

Solution steps

1 Establish how many drops are in 1 mL.
2 Calculate how many millilitres need to be delivered every minute to give 1.2 L in 10 hours.
3 Multiply the number of millilitres per minute by the number of drops in each millilitre.

Adult giving set delivers 20 drops per mL

1.2 L in 10 h = (1200 mL ÷ 10) in 1 h = 120 mL in 1 h

120 mL in 1 h = (120 mL ÷ 60) in 1 min = 2 mL in 1 min

2 mL/min = 2 × 20 drops/min = 40 drops/min

Answer: 40 drops/minute

SELF-ASSESSMENT

Now try the self-assessment questions to ensure you have understood this chapter.

Questions

1   Phenytoin can be given orally as a 3–4 mg/kg daily dose. What dose should be given to a 50 kg female who is 1.5 m tall in order to give 3 mg/kg based on:

   a. Actual body weight?

   b. Ideal body weight?

2   The adult dose of drug *x* is 800 mg but there is no recommended paediatric dose. Based on Table 6.2, what dose of drug *x* would you advise for a four month old child, weighing 6.5 kg?

3   Drug *y* can be prescribed based on weight or surface area. Using an appropriate equation, calculate the dose required for a 162 kg male (2 m in height) based on a prescribed dose of 500 mg/m².

4   A patient is prescribed 250 mg frusemide IV. This should not be given more rapidly than 5 mg/min.

   a. What is the minimum time over which this dose can be given?

   b. Rather than administering the drug neat, a pharmacist advises that the frusemide dose should be dissolved in 100 mL of normal saline. What is the maximum rate (mL/min) at which the drug should be administered?

5   A patient is prescribed 80 mmol of potassium, which is to be given using 480 mL of fluid at a rate of 20 mmol/h. If a normal giving set delivers approximately 20 drops per millilitre, calculate the drop rate required, in drops per minute, to administer the potassium.

6   A paediatric giving set (1 mL = 60 drops) is being used to administer 240 mL of saline over 24 hours. What should the drop rate be set at, in drops/minute?

7   An adult patient is given 60 drops per minute of a drug solution which is 20 mg/5 mL. What dose of the drug are they receiving in 1 hour?

8 A patient with diabetes is being controlled by using an IV sliding scale. A syringe pump containing 75 units soluble insulin in 50 mL saline is available. The patient's blood glucose is measured every hour and the insulin dose is adjusted according to the scale below.

Fingerprick glucose concentration mmol/L	IV soluble insulin units/hour
<2	None – give 50 mL 50% w/v dextrose
2.0–6.4	0.5
6.5–8.9	1.0
9.0–10.9	2.0
11–16.9	3.0
17–28	4.0
>28	8.0

If the patient's blood glucose is currently 12.3 mmol/L, what pump rate should be used (in mL/h)?

9 A syringe pump on a ward is delivering dopamine infusion 0.75% w/v at a rate of 4 mL/h to a 50 kg female. What dose in mcg/kg/min is she receiving (to the nearest whole number)?

10 A dobutamine infusion is running at 2 mL/h for a 100 kg male, the syringe contains 240 mg dobutamine in 40 mL normal saline. What increase is necessary in the infusion rate to increase the dose delivered by 0.5 mcg/kg/min?

References

1 Paediatric Formulary Committee. *BNF for Children*. London: BMJ Publishing Group, Royal Pharmaceutical Society of Great Britain, and RCPCH Publications; 2005.

2 Mosteller RD. Simplified calculation of body-surface area. *NEJM*. 1987; **317**: 1098.

3 Tomlin S. *Paediatric formulary*. 7th ed. London: Guy's and St Thomas', King's College and University Lewisham Hospitals; 2005.

7

Clinical pharmacokinetics

By the end of this chapter you should be able to:
- estimate loading dosages
- estimate maintenance dosages
- determine renal function from serum creatinine concentrations.

Definition of terms

Pharmacokinetic calculations are used to increase the likelihood of obtaining drug serum concentrations within a required range. These calculations invariably require the use of equations and therefore it is appropriate to define the common terminology.

Therapeutic window

The therapeutic window is the serum concentration range within which a drug is most likely to be clinically effective and least likely to cause unwanted side-effects. A serum concentration within the 'therapeutic window' does not, however, demonstrate clinical effectiveness. Clinical indicators are always necessary to determine the effectiveness of therapy.

TABLE 7.1 Therapeutic windows for regularly prescribed drugs

Drug	Serum concentration range
Digoxin	1.5–3 mcg/L
Theophylline	10–20 mg/L*
Phenytoin	10–20 mg/L*
Carbamazepine	4–12 mg/L
Gentamicin	4–8 mg/L (peak)

*Theophylline and phenytoin can be effective from 5 mg/L.

The majority of drugs have a wide therapeutic window and consequently close monitoring of the drug's serum concentration is not clinically justified. Drugs such as digoxin, theophylline, gentamicin, carbamazepine and phenytoin all have narrow therapeutic windows (*see* Table 7.1) thus for patients prescribed these drugs it is important to individualise dosages very carefully. Local biochemistry laboratories may use differing values depending on the standardisation of the equipment.

Bioavailability

Bioavailability (F) is the fraction of the drug that reaches the systemic circulation and is expressed as a number from 0 to 1. Drugs that are extensively metabolised in the gut or liver or are poorly absorbed will have reduced bioavailability. The effect of metabolism in the liver is generally described as the 'first pass effect'. A large first pass effect will invariably produce a low oral bioavailability. Similarly, different formulations and routes of administration can significantly affect bioavailability. It is generally accepted that drugs that are parenterally administered, i.e. via injection, have a bioavailability of 1. The approximate bioavailabilities of regularly used formulations of drugs with narrow therapeutic windows are outlined in Table 7.2.

TABLE 7.2 Approximate bioavailability of regularly prescribed formulations

Drug and formulation	F
Digoxin tablets	0.7
Digoxin elixir	0.77
Phenytoin preparations*	1
Carbamazepine tablets (Tegretol)	1.0
Carbamazepine s/r tablets (Tegretol Retard)	0.85
Aminophylline s/r tablets**	1
Theophylline s/r tablets and capsules	1

*Phenytoin capsules and injections consist of the sodium salt, and the salt fraction (S) must be taken into account when determining the amount of phenytoin absorbed. The S value is 0.92 for both preparations.

**Aminophylline is a theophylline salt and consequently the S value must be taken into account when determining the amount of theophylline absorbed. Approximately 80% by weight of aminophylline is theophylline and hence any aminophylline dose must be multiplied by 0.8 to determine the amount of theophylline reaching the systemic circulation.

In summary

Amount of drug reaching systemic circulation = Bioavailability × Salt fraction × Dose administered

= $F \times S \times$ Dose

Example 7.1   What dose of carbamazepine 'slow release' tablets would be required if a patient was changed from a dose of 850 mg of carbamazepine normal release tablets, ensuring the same amount of drug is delivered to the systemic circulation?

Solution steps

1   Calculate the amount of carbamazepine systemically absorbed from normal release tablets.
2   Calculate the dose of the new formulation required to deliver the same amount of carbamazepine to the systemic circulation.

The dose of carbamazepine systemically absorbed by the patient from the normal release tablets is:

$F \times S \times$ Oral dose = Amount systemically absorbed

$1 \times 1 \times 850$ mg = 850 mg absorbed

Therefore 850 mg must be systemically absorbed from the slow release tablets.

Rearranging the above equation gives:

$$\text{Oral dose} = \frac{\text{Amount systemically absorbed}}{F \times S}$$

$$\text{Oral dose} = \frac{850 \text{ mg}}{0.85 \times 1}$$

Oral dose of slow release tablets = 1000 mg as this would provide a systemic dose of 850 mg.

Answer: 1000 milligrams

Volume of distribution

When a drug has been delivered into the systemic circulation its distribution around the body depends on its lipid and water solubility. Hence the final drug concentration in different tissues will vary. The serum concentration of a drug is most commonly quoted.

The volume of distribution (V_d), used in pharmacokinetic calculations, is the theoretical volume that would be needed to distribute a drug, if it was found at the same concentration throughout the body as that measured in the serum. For example, if a patient has a measured drug serum concentration (C) of 15 mg/L and we know that 300 mg had been systemically absorbed, the volume of distribution would be 20 L, i.e. 20 L of serum would be needed to distribute the dose (300 mg ÷ 15 mg/L = 20 L).

So,

$$\text{Volume of distribution} = \frac{\text{Amount of drug systemically absorbed}}{\text{Serum concentration}}$$

But as we know that:

Amount systemically absorbed = $F \times S \times$ Dose

$$\frac{F \times S \times \text{Dose}}{C}$$

The time at which a serum concentration is measured is important if the drug does not immediately distribute itself between the serum and body tissues. If a drug is initially predominantly distributed in the serum, a serum concentration taken too soon after administration will produce an artificially high result and the V_d will be calculated as being smaller than the actual value. Drugs undergoing this type of distribution, e.g. digoxin, are described as distributing via a two compartment model. A digoxin serum concentration should be measured within six hours after dosing to accurately calculate a patient's V_d.

The population average volumes of distribution per kilogram of actual body weight (ABW) for drugs with a narrow therapeutic index are provided in Table 7.3.

TABLE 7.3 Population volumes of distribution for regularly prescribed drugs

Drug	Volume of distribution (L/kg)
Digoxin	7.3*
Theophylline	0.5
Phenytoin	0.65
Carbamazepine	1.4
Gentamicin	0.25

*Based upon ideal or actual body weight, whichever is lower.

Elimination half-life

This is the time it takes for a drug serum concentration to reduce by half after the drug has been delivered into the systemic circulation. Table 7.4 gives the average elimination half-life ($T_{0.5}$) of commonly prescribed drugs with a narrow therapeutic window. This information is especially useful for determining how many days to withdraw a drug when an overdose is detected. For example, in the case of a drug with $T_{0.5}$ = 12 h it would take 24 hours for the serum concentration to reduce from 20 mg/L to 5 mg/L. This is because after 12 hours the serum concentration will be 10 mg/L and after a further 12 hours it will be 5 mg/L.

TABLE 7.4 Approximate $T_{0.5}$ values for regularly prescribed drugs

Drug	$T_{0.5}$
Digoxin	48 hours
Theophylline	8 hours
Phenytoin	22 hours*
Carbamazepine	30–35 hours

*The half-life of phenytoin is dependent on the serum concentration and consequently this value can vary.

Example 7.2   Roughly how long should a patient's digoxin tablets be stopped if they had a detected serum concentration of 4.6 mcg/L if you wanted to get them back into normal range?

Normal range for digoxin is 1–2 mcg/L

After 48 hours this patient's serum concentration would be 2.3 mcg/L
After a further 48 hours this would be reduced to 1.15mcg/L

Answer: somewhere between 48 and 96 hours

Clearance

Clearance is the volume of serum that is cleared of a drug over a set period of time and is usually expressed in litres per hour. Clearance does not tell you the exact amount of drug cleared, because this is dependent on the drug's serum concentration.

Example 7.3   If a drug has a clearance of 2 L/h, how much will be removed from the body in 24 hours if:

a. The serum concentration is 4 mg/L?

b. The serum concentration is 1 mg/L?

Solution steps

1   Multiply the volume cleared per hour by the serum concentration to determine the total amount of drug cleared in 1 hour.

2   Multiply the total amount of drug cleared in 1 hour by 24 hours.

a. If 2 L of serum are cleared each hour and every litre of serum has 4 mg of drug in it then 8 mg will be cleared each hour.

Amount of drug removed in 24 h will be 8 mg/h × 24 h = 192 mg.

Answer: 192 milligrams

b. If 2 L of serum are cleared each hour and every litre has 1 mg of drug in it then 2 mg will be cleared each hour.

Amount of drug removed in 24 h will be 2 mg/h × 24 h = 48 mg.

Answer: 48 milligrams

Table 7.5 summarises the average clearance values for drugs with small therapeutic windows. Individual patient clearances can be estimated from population values provided in Table 7.5, by multiplying by the actual body weight of the patient. The clearance of digoxin, phenytoin and gentamicin are dependent on other factors and the calculation of these is provided on pages 79–82.

TABLE 7.5 Population 'clearance' for theophylline and carbamazepine

Drug	Clearance L/hr/kg
Theophylline	0.04
Carbamazepine	0.064

Because digoxin and gentamicin are predominantly removed by the kidneys, prior calculation of renal function is necessary to estimate the drug clearance.

Creatinine clearance

Creatinine clearance (Cl_{cr}) is the most practical and accurate measure of renal function and is most easily determined using serum creatinine concentrations. Because serum creatinine concentrations are not independent of age, sex or weight these must be taken into account when calculating creatinine clearance. The equations for calculating creatinine clearance (measured in mL/min) in males and females are as follows:

■ Males

$$Cl_{cr}(mL/min) = \frac{1.23\,(140 - Age)(Weight\ in\ kg)}{Serum\ Creatinine\ \mu mol/L}$$

■ Females

$$Cl_{cr}(mL/min) = \frac{1.04\,(140 - Age)(Weight\ in\ kg)}{Serum\ Creatinine\ \mu mol/L}$$

Because creatinine is a by-product of muscle metabolism, either the patient's ideal body weight (IBW, *see* Chapter 6) or ABW, whichever is lower, should be used.

Once a creatinine clearance has been calculated, the degree of renal impairment can be estimated using the following guidelines:

Cl_{cr}	< 10 mL/min	Severe renal impairment
Cl_{cr}	10–20 mL/min	Moderate renal impairment
Cl_{cr}	> 20 mL/min and < 50 mL/min	Mild renal impairment

Example 7.4   Calculate the renal function of Mrs AS, a 75-year-old patient, who is 1.6 m tall, weighs 65 kg and has a measured serum creatinine of 130 μmol/L

Solution steps
1   Calculate the patient's ideal body weight (IBW).
2   Place either the IBW or ABW, whichever is the lower, into the equation for determining creatinine clearance for females.
3   Use the clearance value obtained to determine the degree of renal impairment.

First, we need to calculate the IBW for a female:

IBW (female) = $0.9H - 92 = (0.9 \times 160 \text{ cm}) - 92 = 52$ kg

ABW = 65 kg

The weight used in the equation is therefore 52 kg.

$$Cl_{cr} \text{ (Females)} = \frac{1.04 \,(140 - 75)(52)}{\text{Serum Creatinine μmol/L}} \text{ mL/min}$$

$$Cl_{cr} \text{ (Females)} = \frac{1.04 \,(140 - 75)(52)}{130 \text{ μmol/L}} \text{ mL/min}$$

$Cl_{cr} = 27$ mL/min

We can therefore assume that this patient has mild renal impairment.

Digoxin clearance

Digoxin clearance is calculated by summing the renal and metabolic clearance of the drug. Renal clearance of digoxin is approximately equal to creatinine clearance and metabolic clearance can be estimated, although it is dependent on whether the patient has congestive heart failure. The presence of congestive heart failure can reduce metabolic and renal clearance of digoxin by 50% and 10%, respectively.

In a patient without heart failure:

Digoxin clearance (mL/min) = $(0.8 \times$ Weight in kg$) + Cl_{cr}$

In a patient with congestive heart failure:

Digoxin clearance (mL/min) = $(0.33 \times$ Weight in kg$) + (0.9 \times Cl_{cr})$

Example 7.5   Estimate the digoxin clearance of Mrs AS, who has an estimated creatinine clearance of 27 mL/min and weighs 65 kg. Assume that Mrs AS does not have congestive heart failure

Solution step

1   Place the values provided into the equation for digoxin clearance for a patient without congestive heart failure.

Digoxin clearance (mL/min) = $(0.8 \times$ Weight in kg$) + Cl_{cr}$

Digoxin clearance (mL/min) = $(0.8 \times 65) + 27$

Digoxin clearance = 79 mL/min

Answer: 79 millilitres/minute

Gentamicin clearance

Gentamicin is almost entirely renally excreted. Consequently, creatinine clearance and gentamicin clearance are the same, unless renal function is markedly diminished. In this instance, the non-renal clearance of 0.0021 L/h/kg is used to estimate gentamicin clearance.

Phenytoin clearance

Phenytoin metabolism is capacity limited, meaning that when the amount of phenytoin entering the body passes a certain point the metabolism of the drug cannot increase accordingly. Consequently, increases in dosage can lead to disproportionate increases in serum concentration.

The metabolism of phenytoin follows the pattern proposed by Michaelis and Menten, and the variables V_m and K_m are used to describe phenytoin pharmacokinetics.

- V_m is the maximum metabolic capacity (mg/kg/day)
- K_m is the plasma concentration at which the rate of metabolism is half the maximum (mg/L)

Using the Michaelis Menten model, phenytoin clearance is calculated from the equation:

$$\text{Clearance of Phenytoin } (Cl_{\text{phenytoin}}) = \frac{V_m}{K_m + \text{Serum concentration (mg/L)}}$$

Example 7.6   Assuming that V_m is 7 mg/kg/day and K_m is 4 mg/L, calculate phenytoin clearance in a 60 kg patient with a serum concentration of 15 mg/L

Solution step

1   Place the values provided into the equation for the clearance of phenytoin.

$$\text{Clearance of Phenytoin } (Cl_{\text{phenytoin}}) = \frac{V_m}{K_m + \text{Serum concentration (mg/L)}}$$

$$\text{Clearance of Phenytoin } (Cl_{\text{phenytoin}}) = \frac{7 \text{ mg/kg/day} \times 60 \text{ kg}}{4 \text{ mg/L} + 15 \text{ mg/L}}$$

$$\text{Clearance of Phenytoin } (Cl_{\text{phenytoin}}) = 22.1 \text{ L/day}$$

In practice, K_m can usually be assumed to be 4 mg/L, and for initial estimates, V_m may be taken as 7 mg/kg/day. However, the value for V_m should always be revised after the first serum concentration has been measured. In order to calculate a revised V_m the following equation should be used:

$$V_m = \frac{(S)(F)(\text{Daily Dose in mg})(K_m + \text{Serum concentration})}{\text{Serum concentration}}$$

This equation can also be rearranged to calculate maintenance dosages:

$$\text{Maintenance dose (mg)} = \frac{(V_m)(\text{Serum concentration})}{(S)(F)(K_m + \text{Serum concentration})}$$

Example 7.7   Estimate the phenytoin maintenance dosage for a 60 kg patient requiring a serum concentration of 15 mg/L. Assume that K_m is 4 mg/L and V_m is 7 mg/kg/day and the patient is to receive capsules

Solution step
1   Place the values provided into the equation for estimating phenytoin maintenance dosages.

From previous information we know that:

Bioavailability (*F*)   = 1

Salt fraction (*S*)   = 0.92

K_m = 4 mg/L

V_m = 7 mg/kg/day

$$\text{Maintenance dose (mg)} = \frac{(V_m)(\text{Serum concentration})}{(S)(F)(K_m + \text{Serum concentration})}$$

$$\text{Maintenance dose (mg)} = \frac{(7 \times 60)(15)}{(0.92)(1)(4+15)}$$

Answer: maintenance dose = 360 mg phenytoin sodium capsules (350 mg in practice)

Example 7.8   After prescribing 350 mg of phenytoin sodium capsules for 5 days to a 60 kg patient the measured serum concentration is 10 mg/L. What dose would be necessary to provide a serum concentration of 15 mg/L?

Solution steps

1   Determine V_m using the serum concentration and dose provided.
2   Estimate phenytoin maintenance dosage with the new V_m.

From previous information we know that:

Bioavailability (F) $= 1$

Salt fraction (S) $= 0.92$

K_m $= 4$ mg/L

$$\text{Maintenance dose (mg)} = \frac{(V_m)(\text{Serum concentration})}{(S)(F)(K_m + \text{Serum concentration})}$$

First, we need to calculate V_m

$$V_m = \frac{(S)(F)(\text{Daily Dose mg})(K_m \text{ Serum concentration})}{\text{Serum concentration}}$$

$$V_m = \frac{(0.92)(1)(350 \text{ mg})(4+10)}{10}$$

$V_m = 450.8$ mg/day (note the patient's weight is already accounted for in the units).

$$\text{Maintenance dose (mg)} = \frac{(V_m)(\text{Serum concentration})}{(S)(F)(K_m + \text{Serum concentration})}$$

$$\text{Maintenance dose (mg)} = \frac{(450.8)(15)}{(1)(0.92)(4+15)}$$

Answer: maintenance dose $= 386.8$ mg phenytoin sodium capsules (400 mg in practice)

Loading dose

If we can estimate a patient's volume of distribution and know the target concentration required, it is possible to estimate an individual patient's loading dose. The amount of drug in the body will be the target serum concentration multiplied by the volume of distribution. The loading dose will then be equal to the amount of drug in the body divided by the bioavailability and salt fraction of the equation used.

Amount of drug in the body = Target conc. (C) × Volume of distribution (V_d)

$$\text{Loading dose} = \frac{\text{Amount of drug in the body}}{\text{Bioavailability } (F) \times \text{Salt fraction } (S)}$$

Substituting,

$$\text{Loading dose} = \frac{C \times V_d}{F \times S}$$

Example 7.9   It is decided that Mrs Jones requires digoxin therapy. She is 60 kg in weight. What oral loading dose would you recommend?

Solution steps

1   Calculate the patient's volume of distribution.
2   Use the equation for loading dose to determine the required dosage.

From previous information we know that:

F = 0.7

V_d = 7.3 L/kg

C = 1.5 mcg/L

This patient's volume of distribution is therefore:

7.3 L/kg × 60 kg = 438 L

$$\text{Loading dose} = \frac{C \times V_d}{F \times S}$$

$$\text{Loading dose} = \frac{1.5 \text{ mcg/L} \times 438 \text{ L}}{0.7 \times 1}$$

Answer: loading dose = 938.6 micrograms

In practice the prescriber would give 1000 mcg as an oral dose.

Example 7.10 What dose of gentamicin would be required to achieve a target concentration of 6 mg/L in an 80 kg woman?

Solution steps
1 Calculate the patient's volume of distribution.
2 Use the equation for loading dose to determine the required dosage.

From previous information we know that:

F = 1

S = 1

V_d = 0.25 L/kg

C = 6 mg/L

This patient's volume of distribution is therefore:

0.25 L/kg × 80 kg = 20 L

$$\text{Required dose} = \frac{V_d \times C}{F \times S}$$

Required dose $= 120$ mg

$$\text{Required dose} = \frac{20\,\text{L} \times 6\,\text{mg/L}}{1 \times 1}$$

Answer: 120 milligrams

One of the assumptions of using the above equation for estimating loading dosages is that during the time taken for the drug to be systemically absorbed there is very little elimination from the body. This assumption generally holds true if elimination of the drug is slow, i.e. it has a long half-life, or if its absorption is rapid. Because gentamicin has a relatively short half-life, the validity of the above equation is dependent on the rate of infusion. In general, if the infusion time is less than one quarter of the half-life (gentamicin $T_{0.5} = 2\text{–}3$ hours), the above equation can be used. Equations to determine the loading dose of gentamicin, which take into account elimination of the drug, are beyond the remit of this book.

Maintenance dosages

The amount of drug required to keep a steady serum concentration is the maintenance dose. By multiplying the drug clearance by the required serum concentration we can calculate how drug is removed, and therefore the amount required to replace it.

Amount of drug removed $= Cl \times C$

$$\text{Maintenance dose} = \frac{\text{Amount of drug removed}}{F \times S}$$

$$\text{Maintenance dose (mg/hr)} = \frac{Cl \times C}{F \times S}$$

$$\text{Maintenance dose every } \tau \text{ hours} = \frac{Cl \times C \times \tau}{F \times S}$$

Example 7.11 What maintenance dose would you recommend, to be given every six hours, if a drug has a clearance of 5 L/h and a serum concentration of 15 mg/L? (Assume $F = 1$ and $S = 1$)

Solution step

1 Use the equation for maintenance dosage.

$$\text{Maintenance dose} = \frac{\text{Clearance (L/hr)} \times \text{Concentration (mg/L)} \times \tau}{\text{Bioavailability } (F) \times \text{Salt fraction } (S)}$$

$$\text{Maintenance dose} = \frac{5 \text{ L/hr} \times 15 \text{ mg/L} \times 6}{1 \times 1}$$

Answer: maintenance dose = 450 milligrams every 6 hours

Example 7.12 Calculate the required daily digoxin maintenance dose for an 80 kg, 75-year-old male patient (1.9 m tall), with a serum creatinine of 210 μmol/L and no heart failure. The required serum concentration is 1.5 mcg/L.

Solution steps

1 Calculate the patient's ideal body weight (IBW).
2 Determine the patient's renal function using either the IBW or ABW, whichever is the lower.
3 Calculate the patient's digoxin clearance.
4 Calculate the required maintenance dose.

From previous information we know that:

F = 0.7 for digoxin tablets

S = 1

C = 1.5 mcg/L

τ = 24 hours

First, we need to calculate the patient's ideal body weight.

IBW (male) = $0.9H - 88 = (0.9 \times 190) - 88 = 83$ kg

In this case the weight to be used is the patient's own weight. Next we need to determine the patient's renal function.

$$Cl_{cr} \text{ (Males)} = \frac{1.23(140 - \text{Age})(\text{Weight in kg})}{\text{Serum creatinine } \mu\text{mol/L}}$$

$$Cl_{cr} \text{ (Males)} = \frac{1.23(140 - 75)(80)}{210}$$

$Cl_{cr} = 30.4$ mL/min (mild renal impairment)

Next we need to determine the digoxin clearance.

Digoxin clearance (mL/min) = $(0.8 \times \text{Weight kg}) + Cl_{cr}$

Digoxin clearance (mL/min) = $64 + 30.4 = 94.4$ mL/min = 5.7 L/h

Finally, we can calculate the recommended maintenance dose.

$$\text{Maintenance dose} = \frac{V_d \times C \times \tau}{F \times S}$$

$$\text{Maintenance dose} = \frac{5.7 \text{ (L/hr)} \times 1.5 \text{ (mcg/L)} \times 24}{0.7 \times 1}$$

Answer: maintenance dose = 293 micrograms daily (250 mcg in practice)

SELF-ASSESSMENT

Now try the self-assessment questions to ensure you have understood this chapter.

Questions

For each of the following questions you may use the previously stated population values.

1   After giving a patient 1200 mg of carbamazepine tablets (normal release) a peak serum concentration of 12 mg/L was measured. Estimate the patient's volume of distribution.

2   100 mcg of a new drug formulation was given to a patient and a total of 85 mcg was recovered in the urine. Calculate the bioavailability of the drug, assuming that it is totally renally excreted.

3   A patient presents in casualty with a peak theophylline serum concentration of 30 mg/L. How long will it take for the serum concentration to reach 7.5 mg/L if they take no further doses?

4   Estimate the renal impairment of a 55 kg, 80-year-old male (1.6 m tall) with a serum creatinine of 180 µmol/L.

5   What loading dose of IV digoxin would you recommend for a 60 kg patient requiring a serum concentration of 1.5 mcg/L?

6   What loading dose of IV aminophylline would you recommend for a 65 kg patient requiring a serum concentration of 10 mg/L?

7   Estimate the gentamicin serum concentration (mg/L) that would be expected 1 hour after a rapidly absorbed infusion of 100 mg had been started. Assume that there had been negligible elimination after 1 hour.

8   What daily maintenance dose of digoxin would you recommend for a 75-year-old, 55 kg female (1.6 m tall) with congestive heart failure and a measured serum creatinine of 170 µmol/L?

9 A 55 kg patient prescribed 300 mg of phenytoin capsules daily has a measured serum concentration of 8 mg/L. What dosage of phenytoin would you recommend in order to obtain a serum concentration of 12 mg/L?

10 What twice-daily maintenance dose of carbamazepine (slow-release tablets) would you recommend for a 70 kg male, if the target concentration was 10 mg/L?

8

Suppository calculations

Suppositories

Suppositories are dosage forms prepared for drug delivery via the rectum. They consist of an active medicament dispersed throughout an inactive base. The bases used in these products can be broadly classified into two groups:

■ Fatty bases. These may be of natural origin, such as theobroma oil (cocoa butter), or synthetic fats such as Witepsol.

■ Hydrophilic bases. The most commonly used hydrophilic base is composed of a solid glycerol/gelatin mixture.

Displacement values

Suppositories are prepared by dissolving or dispersing an active medicament in a molten base and pouring the mixture into a suppository mould. Suppository moulds are normally available in 1 g, 2 g and 4 g sizes – the approximate weights of theobroma oil suppositories that are produced from them – although the volume of the suppository mould will be constant. However, because the density of the medicament may vary considerably from that of the base, the weight of the base required to make a suppository will vary depending on the medicament used. For example, 2 g of a medicament with twice the density of theobroma oil would occupy approximately the same volume as 1 g of the suppository base. The displacement values (DVs) of medicaments are required when calculating the weight of suppository base required to prepare medicated suppositories (see Example 8.1). The displacement value of a medicament is the number of parts, by weight, of a medicament that will displace one part of suppository base (normally theobroma oil). Displacement values for various medicaments are given in the *Pharmaceutical Codex*.

(*Note:* The following examples take no account of preparation losses and it is normal practice to prepare for an excess quantity of suppositories.)

Example 8.1   Calculate the quantities required to make 10 theobroma oil suppositories (2 g mould) each containing 400 mg of zinc oxide (Displacement value = 4.7)

Solution steps

1 Calculate the total weight of zinc oxide required.
2 Calculate what weight of base would be required to prepare 10 unmedicated suppositories.
3 Determine what weight of base would be displaced by the medicament.
4 Calculate, therefore, the weight of base required to prepare the medicated suppositories.

Total weight of zinc oxide required = 400 mg × 10 = 4 g

Weight of base required for unmedicated suppositories = 2 g × 10 = 20 g

As the displacement value of zinc oxide = 4.7

This means that 4.7 g of zinc oxide would displace 1 g of theobroma oil

1 g of zinc oxide would displace 1 ÷ 4.7 g of theobroma oil

So, 4 g of zinc oxide will displace (4 × 1) ÷ 4.7 g of theobroma oil = 0.85 g

Therefore, the weight of base required to make medicated suppositories = 20 − 0.85 g = 19.15 g

Answer: 19.15 grams

Note that for theobroma oil suppositories you can calculate the amount of base displaced by the active ingredient by dividing the amount of active ingredient by the displacement value, e.g. 200 mg of a drug with a DV of 4 will displace 200/4 mg or 50 mg of base in each mould.

Glycero-gelatin base has a density 1.2 times greater than theobroma oil. Therefore, a 1 g suppository mould will produce a 1 g theobroma oil suppository, but a 1.2 g glycero-gelatin suppository. This factor must be taken into account in displacement value calculations.

Example 8.2   Calculate the quantities required to make six glycero-gelatin suppositories (4 g mould), each containing 100 mg aminophylline (Displacement value = 1.3)

Solution steps
1   Calculate the total weight of aminophylline required.
2   Calculate what weight of glycero-gelatin base would be required to prepare 10 unmedicated suppositories.
3   Determine what weight of base would be displaced by the medicament.
4   Calculate, therefore, the weight of base required to prepare the medicated suppositories.

Total weight of aminophylline required = 100 mg × 6 = 600 mg or 0.6 g

Weight of base required for unmedicated suppositories = 4 g × 6 × 1.2 (to take account of the greater density of this base) = 28.8 g

As the displacement value of aminophylline = 1.3

This means that 1.3 g of aminophylline displaces 1 g of theobroma oil

So, 1 g of aminophylline displaces 1 ÷ 1.3 g of theobroma oil

0.6 g of aminophylline displace (1 × 0.6) ÷ 1.3 g of theobroma oil = 0.46 g of theobroma oil

This means that the aminophylline would displace 0.46 g × 1.2 of the glycero-gelatin base = 0.55 g

Therefore, the weight of base required to make medicated suppositories = 28.8 g – 0.55 g = 28.25 g

Answer: 28.25 grams

Medicaments included as a percentage w/w

If a medicament is present in a suppository as a percentage w/w, then its displacement value is not required when calculating the respective amounts of medicament and base required to prepare the suppository.

Example 8.3   What quantities are required to prepare eight theobroma oil suppositories, in a 4 g mould, containing 1% w/w lignocaine hydrochloride?

Solution steps

1   Calculate the total weight of the medicated suppositories.
2   Calculate, therefore, the weight of the drug required (1% of the total weight).
3   Subtract the weight of the drug from the total weight of the suppositories to find the weight of the base required.

Total weight of the suppositories = 32 g

Weight of drug required (1% w/w) = (32 × 1) ÷ 100 g = 0.32 g

Therefore, weight of base required = 32 g – 0.32 g = 31.68 g

Answer: 31.68 grams

Again, if a glycero-gelatin base is used, the appropriate correction factor must be used as a 1 g mould for a theobroma oil suppository will actually hold 1.2 g of glycero-gelatin base.

Example 8.4   Prepare 12 glycero-gelatin suppositories, containing 0.5% w/w cinchocaine hydrochloride. Use a 2 g mould

Solution steps

1   Calculate the total weight of the medicated suppositories, allowing for the greater density of the glycero-gelatin base.
2   Calculate the weight of the drug required.
3   Subtract the weight of the drug from the total weight of the suppositories to determine the weight of the base required.

Total weight of the suppositories = 12 × 2 g × 1.2 = 28.8 g

Weight of drug required = (28.8 g × 0.5) ÷ 100 = 0.144 g (or 144 mg)

Therefore weight of base required = 28.8 g – 0.144 g = 28.66 g

Answer: 28.66 grams

SELF-ASSESSMENT

Now try the self-assessment questions to ensure you have understood this chapter.

Questions

1 How would you prepare 10 theobroma oil suppositories (1 g mould) containing 2.5% w/w bismuth subgallate?

2 How would you prepare six theobroma oil suppositories (2 g mould) containing 10% w/w zinc oxide?

3 Six theobroma oil suppositories (2 g), each containing 125 mg of paracetamol, are to be prepared. The displacement value of paracetamol is 1.5. What quantities of base and medicament are required?

4 You are asked to prepare 11 theobroma oil suppositories (2 g mould) each containing 100 mg of aspirin (DV = 1.1). What weights of base and medicament are required?

5 Prepare 10 theobroma oil suppositories, each containing 50 mg of bismuth subgallate (DV = 2.5). If a 2 g mould is used, what quantities of base and medicament are required?

6 A prescriber requests five glycero-gelatin suppositories be made, containing 1% w/w hydrocortisone acetate. If a 4 g mould is used, what quantities of base and medicament are needed?

7 Prepare eight glycero-gelatin suppositories (in a 2 g mould) each containing 20 mg of morphine hydrochloride (DV = 1.6).

8 Ten glycero-gelatin suppositories, each containing 30 mg phenobarbitone sodium (DV = 1.2), are to be prepared using a 1 g mould. What quantities of base and medicament are required?

9 Prepare 12 glycero-gelatin suppositories, in a 2 g mould, each containing 50 mg of diphenhydramine hydrochloride (DV = 1.2).

10 You are required to prepare 10 theobroma oil suppositories (2 g). Each suppository must contain 50 mg of bismuth subgallate (DV = 2.5) and 10 mg of hydrocortisone acetate (DV = 1.5). Calculate the weight of each medicament and of theobroma oil required to prepare the suppositories.

(*Hint:* Calculate the weight of base displaced by each medicament and subtract both these from the weight of the unmedicated suppositories.)

Summary test

Questions

1   Add 0.25 litres, 75 millilitres and 4000 microlitres. Give your answer in millilitres.

2   A patient is prescribed 5 mL of a mixture to be taken four times a day for seven days. How much of the mixture should be supplied?

3   An intravenous infusion contains 40 mmol of potassium chloride. What is the mass of potassium chloride contained in the infusion? (Take RMM of potassium chloride to be 80.)

4   How much salicylic acid is present in 350 g of a cream containing 2% w/w salicylic acid?

5   What volume of a 1:10,000 solution of adrenaline would contain 20 mg of the drug?

6   A patient uses 50 mL of a 1:1000 solution of an antiseptic mouthwash, four times a day, for seven days. How many grams of the antiseptic have been used?

7   How would you prepare 500 mL of Chloral Elixir Paediatric BP?

Chloral Elixir Paediatric BP:

Chloral hydrate	200 mg
Water	0.1 mL
Blackcurrant syrup	1 mL
Syrup	to 5 mL

8   What quantity of each ingredient is required to prepare 150 g of Coal Tar and Zinc Ointment BP?

Coal Tar and Zinc Ointment BP:

Strong coal tar solution	100 g
Zinc oxide	300 g
Yellow soft paraffin	600 g

9 What quantity of each ingredient is required to prepare 400 g of Zinc and Salicylic Acid Paste BP?

Zinc and Salicylic Acid Paste BP:

Zinc oxide	24%
Salicylic acid	2%
Starch	24%
White soft paraffin	50%

10 A patient is directed to use 20 mL of a 1:10,000 solution of potassium permanganate twice a day for 10 days. You have in stock a 4% w/v solution of the compound. How much of the concentrate will you require to dispense the prescription?

11 How many grams of emulsifying ointment must be *added* to 400 g of 2% w/w salicylic acid in emulsifying ointment, in order to reduce the salicylic acid concentration to 0.5% w/w?

12 A prescriber requests that sufficient dextrose be added to 500 mL of a 0.18% w/v sodium chloride infusion to give a final concentration of 4% w/v dextrose. What volume of a 40% w/w dextrose solution should be added to the infusion?

13 An ointment contains 1% w/w calamine. What weight of calamine powder should be added to 200 g of the ointment to produce a 5% w/w calamine ointment?

14 A patient is prescribed 5 mg bumetanide in 500 mL glucose 5% w/v, via IV infusion. This should not be given more rapidly than 100 mcg/min. At what rate (mL/min) should the drug be administered?

15 A syringe pump is delivering dopamine infusion 160 mg/50 mL at a rate of 5 mL/h to an 80 kg male. What dose (in mcg/kg/min) is he receiving?

16 Calculate the renal function of an 80-year-old female patient, who is 1.7 m tall, weighs 60 kg and has a measured serum creatinine of 170 μmol/L.

17 What loading dose would you recommend for a male patient, 80 kg, 1.8 m tall, requiring digoxin orally and a serum concentration of 1.2 mcg/L?

18 What daily maintenance dose of digoxin would you recommend for the same 80 kg, 1.8 m tall male patient (Question 17), with congestive heart failure, a creatinine clearance of 18 mL/min and a required serum concentration of 1.2 mcg/L?

19 Prepare 12 theobroma oil suppositories, each containing 100 mg of bismuth subgallate (take DV = 2.4). If a 4 g mould is used, what quantities of base and medicament are required?

20 A prescriber requests that 10 glycero-gelatin suppositories be made, containing 0.5% w/w hydrocortisone acetate. If a 2 g mould is used, what quantities of base and medicament are needed?

Answers to the self-assessment questions

Chapter 1

1 If we approximate the weight of the ointment to 1000 grams, 30% of that is 300 grams. True answer is 3.03 grams.

2 Approximate weight of ointment to 50 grams, so total amount of ointment is approximately $50 \times 50 = 2500$ grams. True answer is 2400 grams.

3 Fraction is $\frac{25}{125} = \frac{5}{25} = \frac{1}{5}$ (simply by dividing top and bottom by 5). As a percentage $= \frac{100}{5} = 20\%$

4 $\frac{21}{105} = \frac{7}{35} =$ (divide by 3 top and bottom) $= \frac{1}{5} = 0.2$

5 $22\% = \frac{22}{100} = 0.22$

6 $\frac{18}{4} = \frac{9}{2} = 4.5$

7 $\frac{0.12}{0.3} = \frac{1.2}{3} = \frac{12}{30} = \frac{6}{15} = \frac{2}{5} = 0.4$

8 $\frac{2}{18} = \frac{1}{9} = 0.111\%$

9 $PV = nRT$ so $nR = \frac{PV}{T}$ so $n = \frac{PV}{RT}$

10 $\frac{b^2 + 4ac}{2a}$

   Multiply both sides by $2a$ so, $2ax = b^2 + 4ac$

   Subtract b^2 from both sides so, $2ax - b^2 = 4ac$

   Divide both sides by $4a$ so, $c = \frac{2ax - b^2}{4a}$

Chapter 2

1   7 kg $= 7000$ g
    75 g $= 75$ g
    750,000 mcg $= 750$ mg $= 0.75$ g
    Total weight $= 7075.75$ g

2   0.04 L $= 40$ mL
    20 mL $= 20$ mL
    200 µl $= 0.2$ mL
    Total volume $= 60.2$ mL

3   Daily, the patient takes 4×250 mg minocycline $= 1000$ mg $=$
    1 g minocycline. In 20 days, the patient takes 1 g $\times 20 = 20$ g
    minocycline.

4   Weight of chlorpheniramine maleate required:
    4 mg $\times 10,000 = 40,000$ mg $= 40$ g
    Weight of phenylpropanolamine hydrochloride required:
    50 mg $\times 10,000 = 500,000$ mg $= 500$ g

5   Weight of oestradiol required:
    8 mg $\times 50,000 = 400,000$ mg $= 400$ g

6   Weight of salmeterol in each inhaler:
    50 mcg $\times 200 = 10,000$ mcg $= 10$ mg

7   Daily, the patient takes 15 mL $\times 2 = 30$ mL
    In 14 days, the patient will take 30 mL $\times 14 = 420$ mL

8   Weight of sodium bicarbonate taken $= 600$ mg $\times 7 = 4200$ mg
    $= 4.2$ g
    84 g of sodium bicarbonate is equivalent to 1 mol, or 1000 mmol
    1 g of sodium bicarbonate is equivalent to $1000 \div 84$ mmol
    4.2 g of sodium bicarbonate is equivalent to $(1000 \div 84) \times$
        4.2 mmol $= 50$ mmol

9   1 mol of sodium chloride weighs 60 g
    1 mmol of sodium chloride weighs 60 mg
    30 mmol of sodium chloride weighs 60×30 mg $= 1800$ mg $= 1.8$ g

10 60 g of sodium chloride is equivalent to 1 mol
60 mg of sodium chloride is equivalent to 1 mmol
1 mg of sodium chloride is equivalent to 1 ÷ 60 mmol
120 mg of sodium chloride is equivalent to (1 ÷ 60) × 120 mmol
  = 2 mmol

75 g of potassium chloride is equivalent to 1 mol
75 mg of potassium chloride is equivalent to 1 mmol
1 mg of potassium chloride is equivalent 1 ÷ 75 mmol
150 mg of potassium chloride is equivalent to (1 ÷ 75) × 150 mmol
  = 2 mmol

1 mmol of sodium chloride provides 1 mmol of chloride
1 mmol of potassium chloride provides 1 mmol of chloride
Therefore, the total amount of chloride = 2 + 2 mmol = 4 mmol

Chapter 3

1 Each dose contains 2 mg × 10 = 20 mg of drug
Daily, the patient takes 20 mg × 3 = 60 mg of drug
In one week, the patient takes 60 mg × 7 = 420 mg of drug

2 Weight of aspirin dissolved = 300 mg × 2 = 600 mg
600 mg of aspirin are dissolved in 120 mL water
0.6 g of aspirin are dissolved in 120 mL water
(0.6 ÷ 120) g of aspirin are dissolved in 1 mL water
(0.6 ÷ 120) × 100 g of aspirin are dissolved in 100 mL water
  = 0.5 g
0.5 g of aspirin are dissolved in 100 mL water
Therefore, the concentration of the solution is 0.5% w/v

3 0.25 g of the antibiotic are dissolved in 100 mL of the solution
0.25 ÷ 100 g of the antibiotic are dissolved in 1 mL of the solution
(0.25 ÷ 100) × 50 g of the antibiotic are dissolved in 50 mL of
solution = 0.125 g of the antibiotic is required

4 100 mL of the liniment contains 5 mL of methyl salicylate

1 mL of the liniment contains 5 ÷ 100 mL of methyl salicylate

600 mL of the liniment contains (5 × 600) ÷ 100 mL of methyl salicylate

(5 × 600) ÷ 100 mL = 30 mL of methyl salicylate

5 100 g of cream will contain 0.5 g hydrocortisone

1 g of cream will contain 0.5 ÷ 100 g hydrocortisone

120 g of cream will contain (0.5 ÷ 100) × 120 g hydrocortisone = 0.6 g of hydrocortisone

6 0.9 g of sodium chloride are dissolved in 100 mL of the infusion

9 g of sodium chloride are dissolved in 1 L of the infusion

60 g of sodium chloride is the weight of 1 mol or 1000 mmol

1 g of sodium chloride is the weight of 1000 ÷ 60 mmol

9 g of sodium chloride is the weight of (1000 ÷ 60) × 9 mmol
= 9000 ÷ 60 mmol = 15 mmol

So, the solution is 15 mmol/L

7 1 g of adrenaline is dissolved in 20,000 mL of solution

1 mg of adrenaline is dissolved in 20,000 ÷ 1000 mL of solution
= 20 mL

50 mg of adrenaline is dissolved in 20 × 50 mL = 1000 mL = 1 L

8 1 mol of sodium bicarbonate weighs 84 g

1000 mmol of sodium bicarbonate weighs 84 g

Hence, in the solution, 84 g of sodium bicarbonate are dissolved in 1000 mL

Therefore, 8.4 g are dissolved in 100 mL of the solution

So, the concentration of the solution is 8.4% w/v

9 1 g of antiseptic is dissolved in 8000 mL of the solution

1 ÷ 8000 g of the antiseptic is dissolved in 1 mL of the solution

(1 ÷ 8000) × 200 g of the antiseptic is dissolved in 200 mL of the solution

So, daily the patient uses $(1 \div 8000) \times 200$ g of the antiseptic
$= 0.025$ g
In 10 days, the patient uses 0.025 g $\times 10 = 0.25$ g of the antiseptic.

10 First, calculate how much anhydrous drug is required to prepare the solution.

4 g of the anhydrous drug must be dissolved in 100 mL of solution.

$4 \div 100$ g of the anhydrous drug must be dissolved in 1 mL of solution.

$(4 \div 100) \times 5000$ g of the anhydrous drug must be dissolved in 5000 mL of solution $= 200$ g of anhydrous drug required.

However, the drug powder contains 10% w/w moisture; therefore: 90% w/w of the powder is the anhydrous drug.

So, 200 g of the anhydrous drug represents 90% of the weight of the powder required.

Therefore, the total weight of powder required $= (200 \div 90) \times 100$ g $= (2000 \div 9)$ g $= 222.2$ g

Chapter 4

1 Prepare 250 mL of Acid Gentian Mixture BP

Concentrated compound gentian infusion	100 mL	25 mL
Dilute hydrochloric acid	50 mL	12.5 mL
Double strength chloroform water	500 mL	125 mL
Water	to 1000 mL	to 250 mL

2 Prepare 150 mL of Potassium Citrate Mixture BP

Potassium citrate	300 g	45 g
Citric acid monohydrate	50 g	7.5 g
Lemon spirit	5 mL	0.75 mL
Quillaia tincture	10 mL	1.5 mL
Syrup	250 mL	37.5 mL
Double strength chloroform water	300 mL	45 mL
Water	to 1000 mL	to 150 mL

3 Prepare 300 mL of Chloral Elixir Paediatric BP

Chloral hydrate	200 mg	12 g
Water	0.1 mL	6 mL
Blackcurrant syrup	1 mL	60 mL
Syrup	to 5 mL	to 300 mL

4 Prepare 200 mL of Paediatric Ferrous Sulphate Mixture BP

Ferrous sulphate	60 mg	2.4 g
Ascorbic acid	10 mg	400 mg
Orange syrup	0.5 mL	20 mL
Double strength chloroform water	2.5 mL	100 mL
Water	to 5 mL	to 200 mL

5 What quantities of each ingredient are required to prepare 50 g of Coal Tar and Zinc Ointment BP?

Strong coal tar solution	100 g	5 g
Zinc oxide	300 g	15 g
Yellow soft paraffin	600 g	30 g

6 What quantity of each ingredient is required to prepare 600g of Zinc and Salicylic Acid Paste BP?

Zinc oxide	24%	144 g
Salicylic acid	2%	12 g
Starch	24%	144 g
White soft paraffin	50%	300 g

7 Prepare 20,000 mL of Magnesium Hydroxide Mixture BP

Magnesium sulphate	47.5 g	950 g
Sodium hydroxide	15 g	300 g
Light magnesium oxide	52.5 g	1050 g
Chloroform	2.5 mL	50 mL
Water	to 1000 mL	to 20,000 mL

8 Prepare 30 g of the following ointment

Fluocinolone acetonide cream	10%	3 g
Aqueous cream	to 100%	to 30 g (i.e. 27 g)

9 Prepare 75 g of the following cream

| Betamethasone cream | 1 part | 15 g |
| Aqueous cream | 4 parts | 60 g |

10 Prepare 80 g of the following ointment

| Dithranol ointment | 1 part | 20 g |
| White soft paraffin | to | 4 parts to 80 g (i.e. 60 g) |

(*Note:* The second line of this formula states 'to 4 parts', indicating that white soft paraffin must comprise three parts of the ointment.)

Chapter 5

1 Use the formula $C_1 \times V_1 = C_2 \times V_2$

$C_1 = 0.2\%$ w/v

$V_1 = ?$

C_2 is a 1:5000 solution $= 0.02\%$ w/v

$V_2 = 1\,L = 1000\,mL$

$0.2 \times V_1 = 0.02 \times 1000$

$V_1 = (0.02 \times 1000) \div 0.2 = 100\,mL$

2 Again, use $C_1 \times V_1 = C_2 \times V_2$

$C_1 = 4\%$ w/v

$V_1 = 100\,mL$

C_2 is a 1:5000 solution $= 0.02\%$ w/v

$V_2 = ?$

$4 \times 100 = 0.02 \times V_2$

$V_2 = (4 \times 100) \div 0.02 = 20,000\,mL = 20\,L$

3 Determine what volume of the dilute solution the patient requires

Daily the patient uses $50\,mL \times 2 = 100\,mL$

In five days, the patient uses $100\,mL \times 5 = 500\,mL$

Now use $C_1 \times V_1 = C_2 \times V_2$

$C_1 = 2\%$ w/v

$V_1 = ?$

C_2 is a 1:10,000 solution of potassium permanganate = 0.01% w/v

$V_2 = 500$ mL

$2 \times V_1 = 0.01 \times 500$

$V_1 = (0.01 \times 500) \div 2 = 2.5$ mL

4 $C_1 \times V_1 = C_2 \times V_2$

$C_1 = 13\%$ w/v

$V_1 = 50$ mL

$C_2 = 0.65\%$ w/v

$V_2 = ?$

$13 \times 50 = 0.65 \times V_2$

$V_2 = (13 \times 50) \div 0.65 = 1000$ mL

Therefore, to carry out the dilution, we must *add* 950 mL to the solution.

5 Use $C_1 \times M_1 = C_2 \times M_2$

$C_1 = 5\%$ w/w

$M_1 = 200$ g

$C_2 = 2\%$ w/w

$M_2 = ?$

$5 \times 200 = 2 \times M_2$

$M_2 = (5 \times 200) \div 2 = 500$ g

Therefore, to carry out the dilution, we must add $500 - 200 = 300$ g of emulsifying ointment.

6 $\dfrac{\text{Initial weight of drug} + \text{added weight of drug}}{\text{Initial volume of solution} + \text{added volume of solution}} = \dfrac{5}{100}$

$\dfrac{0 + x}{1000 + \frac{100x}{25}} = \dfrac{5}{100}$

$5000 + 20x = 100x$

$5000 = 80x$

$x = (500 \div 8)$ g

$x = 62.5$ g

62.5 g of dextrose are dissolved in $(100 \times 62.5) \div 25$ mL of the 25% w/v solution = 250 mL

7   The final concentration required is 40 mmol/L

    1 mol of potassium weighs 40 g

    1 mmol of potassium weighs 40 ÷ 1000 g

    40 mmol of potassium weighs (40 ÷ 1000) × 40 g = 1.6 g

    Therefore, the final concentration required is 1.6 g/L, or 0.16 g/100 mL = 0.16% w/v potassium chloride.

$$\frac{\text{Initial weight of drug} + \text{added weight of drug}}{\text{Initial volume of solution} + \text{added volume of solution}} = \frac{0.16}{100}$$

    Initial weight of drug = 0 g

    Added weight of drug = x g

    Initial volume of solution = 1000 mL

    Added volume of solution = (100 ÷ 16) x g

$$\frac{0 + x}{1000 + \frac{100x}{16}} = \frac{0.16}{100}$$

    $100x = 160 + x$

    $99x = 160$

    $x = 1.6$ grams

    This weight of potassium chloride is dissolved in (100 ÷ 16) × 1.6 mL = 10 mL

    Therefore 10 mL of the potassium chloride solution should be added to the bag.

8   $\dfrac{\text{Initial weight of drug} + \text{added weight of drug}}{\text{Initial weight of cream} + \text{added weight of drug}} = \dfrac{1}{100}$

    Initial weight of drug = 0.03 g (since we have 30 g of a 0.1% w/w cream)

    Added weight of drug = x g

    Initial weight of cream = 30 g

$$\frac{0.03 + x}{30 + x} = \frac{1}{100}$$

    $100(0.03 + x) = 30 + x$

    $3 + 100x = 30 + x$

    $99x = 27$

    $11x = 3$

    $x = 0.27$ g

9 Use the same formula as the previous question.

Initial weight of drug = 1 g (as we have 50 g of a 2% w/w ointment)

Added weight of drug = x g

Initial weight of ointment = 50 g

$$\frac{1+x}{50+x} = \frac{10}{100}$$

$100(1 + x) = 10(50 + x)$

$100 + 100x = 500 + 10x$

$90x = 400$

$9x = 40$

$x = 4.44$ g

10 The same formula can be used here as in the previous two questions; however, the unknown quantities are different. The initial weight of the 10% w/w ointment is unknown, but this must be made up to 30 g with the active ingredient.

Let the initial weight of the cream = x g

Initial weight of drug = x/10 g, or 0.1x g (since the initial cream contains 10% w/w coal tar solution)

Added weight of drug = (30 − x) g (since the final weight of the cream is to be 30 g)

Substituting into the equation:

$$\frac{0.1x + (30 - x)}{x + (30 - x)} = \frac{12}{100}$$

Thus:

$$\frac{30 - 0.9x}{30} = \frac{12}{100}$$

$100(30 − 0.9x) = 360$

$3000 − 90x = 360$

$90x = 2640$

$9x = 264$

$x = 29.33$ g

Therefore, the initial weight of cream to be used = 29.33 g and 0.66 g of coal tar solution must be added to produce 30 g of a 12% w/w ointment.

Chapter 6

1   a. If the ABW = 50 kg and dose is 3 mg/kg, amount required is
        $50 \times 3 = 150$ mg

    b. IBW = $(0.9 \times 150) - 92 = 135 - 92 = 43$ kg
        If the dose is 3 mg/kg, $43 \times 3 = 129$ mg

2   From Table 6.2 the dose should be 20% of the adult dose
    10% of 800 mg = 80 mg and therefore 20% = 160 mg

3   $\sqrt{\frac{H \times W}{3600}} = \sqrt{\frac{162 \times 200}{3600}}$
    BSA = 3 m², dose is 500 mg/m² and therefore 500 mg/m² $\times$ 3 m²
    required = 1500 mg

4   a. If the total amount required is 250 mg and this can be given at
        5 mg/min
        250 mg $\div$ 5 mg/min = 50 minutes

    b. 250 mg in 100 mL = 2.5 mg/mL or 5 mg/2 mL
        Patient requires 5 mg/min = 2 mL/min

5   20 mmol in one hour is one quarter of 80 mmol
    120 mL is one quarter of 480 mL and therefore patient given
        120 mL/h
    120 mL/h = 2 mL/min (120 $\div$ 60)
    1 mL = 20 drops, 2 mL = 40 drops; therefore, drop rate = 40 drops/
        min

6   240 mL per 24 h = 10 mL/h
    10 mL/h $\times$ 60 drops/mL = 600 drops/h or 10 drops/min

7   20 drops = 1 mL
    60 drops = 3 mL
    60 drops/min = 3 mL/min = 180 mL/h (3 $\times$ 60)
    Dose is 20 mg/5 mL = 200 mg/50 mL or 40 mg/10 mL
    180 mL = 3 $\times$ 50 mL + 3 $\times$ 10 mL = 3 $\times$ 200 mg + 3 $\times$ 40 mg
        = 720 mg in 1 hour

8 The concentration of insulin in the syringe pump is 75 units in 50 mL

This is equivalent to 1.5 units/mL

From the table provided a blood glucose of 12.3 mmol/L requires 3 units per hour

3 units can be obtained from 2 mL of the solution in the syringe pump

Pump rate is therefore 2 mL/h

9 0.75% w/v = 0.75 g/100 mL or 750 mg/100 mL or 7.5mg/mL

Patient is receiving 4 mL/h = 4 mL/h × 7.5 mg/mL = 30 mg/h = 30,000 mcg/h

30,000 mcg/h = 500 mcg/min (30,000/60)

She weighs 50 kg and is therefore receiving 10 mcg/kg/min (500/50)

10 240 mg/40 mL = 6 mg/mL

Patient receives 2 mL/h which is equivalent to 12 mg/h

or 12,000 mcg/h or 200 mcg/min

Patient is 100 kg, therefore receiving 2 mcg/kg/min

To increase rate by 0.5 mcg/kg/min need to increase dose by 25%, i.e. from 2 mL/h up to 2.5 mL/h

Chapter 7

1 Bioavailability (F) = 1

Salt fraction (S) = 1

Volume of distribution = $\frac{(F)(S)\text{Dose}}{C}$

Volume of distribution = $\frac{(1)(1)1200 \text{ mg}}{12 \text{ mg/L}}$

Volume of distribution = 100 L

2 Amount of drug reaching systemic circulation = Bioavailability × Salt fraction × Dose administered = $F \times S \times$ Dose

Assuming that amount excreted in the urine represents the amount of systemically absorbed then:

85 mcg $= F \times 1 \times 100$ mcg

$F = 0.85$

3 From previous information the $T_{0.5}$ for theophylline $= 8$ h
Therefore, time taken for serum concentration to fall to one-quarter
its original value will be 16 hours.

4 IBW (male) $= 0.9H - 88 = (0.9 \times 165 \text{ cm}) - 92 = 56.5$ kg
The weight used in the equation is therefore 55 kg.

$$Cl_{cr} = \frac{1.23(140 - \text{Age})(\text{Weight in kg})}{\text{Serum Creatinine } \mu\text{mol/L}}$$

$$Cl_{cr} = \frac{1.23(140 - 80)(55)}{180}$$

$Cl_{cr} = 22.5$ mL/min (mild renal impairment)

5 Bioavailability (F) $= 1$
  Salt fraction (S) $= 1$
  Volume of distribution (V_d) $= 7.3$ L/kg
  Target concentration $= 1.5$ mcg/L

This patient's volume of distribution is therefore:
7.3 L/kg $\times$ 60 kg $= 438$ L

Required dose $= \dfrac{V_d \times C}{F \times S}$

Required dose $= \dfrac{438 \text{ L} \times 1.5 \text{ mcg/L}}{1 \times 1}$

Required dose $= 657$ mcg digoxin injection

6 Bioavailability (F) $= 1$
  Salt fraction (S) $= 0.8$
  Volume of distribution (V_d) $= 0.5$ L/kg
  Target concentration $= 10$ mg/L

This patient's volume of distribution is therefore:
0.5 L/kg $\times$ 65 kg $= 32.5$ L

Required dose $= \dfrac{\text{Volume of distribution } (V_d) \times \text{Concentration } (C)}{\text{Bioavailability } (F) \times \text{Salt fraction } (S)}$

Required dose $= \dfrac{32.5 \times 10}{1 \times 0.8}$

Required dose $= 406.2$ mg aminophylline

7 Bioavailability (F)   = 1
   Salt fraction (S)   = 1
   Volume of distribution (V_d)   = 0.25 L/kg

This patient's volume of distribution is therefore:
0.25 L/kg × 70 kg = 17.5 L

To estimate the concentration the equation for determining loading dosages needs to be rearranged.

$$\text{Required dose} = \frac{\text{Volume of distribution } (V_d) \times \text{Concentration } (C)}{\text{Bioavailability } (F) \times \text{Salt fraction } (S)}$$

$$C = \frac{\text{Dose} \times F \times S}{V_d}$$

$$C = \frac{100 \text{ mg} \times 1 \times 1}{17.5 \text{ L}}$$

$$C = 5.71 \text{ mg/L}$$

8 Bioavailability (F)   = 0.7 for digoxin tablets
   Salt fraction (S)   = 1
   Desired serum concentration (C)   = 1.5 mcg/L

First, calculate the ideal body weight.
IBW (female) = $0.9H - 92$ = 0.9 (160) − 92   = 52 kg

In this case the weight to be used is the IBW. Next, determine the patient's renal function.

$$Cl_{cr} = \frac{1.04(140 - \text{Age})(\text{Weight in Kg})}{\text{Serum creatinine } \mu\text{mol/L}}$$

$$Cl_{cr} \text{ (females)} = \frac{1.04(140 - 75)(52)}{170}$$

Cl_{cr} = 20.7 mL/min (mild renal impairment)

Next, determine the digoxin clearance for a patient with congestive heart failure.
Digoxin clearance (mL/min) = (0.33 × Weight in kg) + (0.9 × Cl_{cr})
Digoxin clearance (mL/min) = (0.33 × 52) + (0.9 × 20.7)
Digoxin clearance (mL/min) = 17.2 + 18.60 = 35.8 mL/min
    = 2.15 L/h

Finally, calculate the recommended maintenance dose.

$$\text{Maintenance dose} = \frac{\text{Clearance (L/hr)} \times \text{Concentration (mg/L)} \times \tau}{\text{Bioavailability }(F) \times \text{Salt fraction }(S)}$$

$$\text{Maintenance dose} = \frac{215 \times 1.5 \times 24}{0.7 \times 1}$$

Maintenance dose = 110.6 mcg daily (125 mcg in practice)

9 Bioavailability (F) = 1

 Salt fraction (S) = 0.92

 K_m = 4 mg/L

First, calculate V_m

$$V_m = \frac{(S)(F)(\text{Daily Dose mg})(K_m + \text{Serum concentration})}{\text{Serum concentration}}$$

$$V_m = \frac{0.92 \times 300 \times (4 + 8)}{8}$$

V_m = 414 mg/day

$$\text{Daily dose (mg)} = \frac{(V_m)(\text{Serum concentration})}{(S)(F)(K_m + \text{Serum concentration})}$$

$$\text{Daily dose (mg)} = \frac{414 \times 12}{1 \times 0.92 \times (4 + 12)}$$

Daily dose (mg) = 337.5 mg phenytoin capsules (350 mg in practice)

10 $F = 0.85$

 $S = 1$

 $C = 10$ mg/L

 $\tau = 12$ h

 $V_d = 0.064$ L/h/kg

Patient's clearance of carbamazepine = 0.064 L/h/kg × 70 kg

 = 4.48 L/h

$$\text{Maintenance dose} = \frac{\text{Clearance (L/hr)} \times \text{Concentration (mg/L)} \times \tau}{\text{Bioavailability }(F) \times \text{Salt fraction }(S)}$$

$$\text{Maintenance dose} = \frac{4.48 \times 10 \times 12}{0.85 \times 1}$$

Maintenance dose = 632 mg every 12 hours (600 mg 12 hourly in practice)

Chapter 8

1. Total weight of the suppositories = 10 g

   Weight of the drug required (2.5% w/w) = (10 × 2.5) ÷ 100 = 0.25 g

   Therefore, the weight of base required = 10 g − 0.25 g = 9.75 g

2. Total weight of the suppositories = 12 g

   Weight of the drug required = (12 × 10) ÷ 100 = 1.2 g

   Therefore, the weight of base required = 12 − 1.2 g = 10.8 g

3. Total weight of medicament required = 6 × 125 mg = 750 mg = 0.75 g

   Weight of base for six unmedicated suppositories = 6 × 2 g = 12 g

   As the displacement value of paracetamol = 1.5, 1.5 g of paracetamol will displace 1 g of theobroma oil, 1 g of paracetamol will displace 1 ÷ 1.5 g of theobroma oil

   Therefore, 0.75 g of paracetamol will displace 0.75 ÷ 1.5 g of theobroma oil = 0.5 g

   Therefore, the weight of base required to make medicated suppositories = 12 g − 0.5 g = 11.5 g

4. Total weight of aspirin required = 11 × 100 mg = 1100 mg = 1.1 g

   Weight of base required for unmedicated suppositories = 11 × 2 g = 22 g

   As the displacement value of aspirin = 1.1,

   1.1 g of aspirin will displace 1 g of theobroma oil,

   Therefore, the weight of base required to make medicated suppositories = 22 g − 1 g = 21 g

5. Weight of bismuth subgallate required = 10 × 50 mg = 500 mg or 0.5 g

   Weight of base required for unmedicated suppositories = 10 × 2 g = 20 g

   As the displacement value of bismuth subgallate = 2.5,

   2.5 g of bismuth subgallate will displace 1 g of theobroma oil,

   1 g of bismuth subgallate will displace 1 ÷ 2.5 g of theobroma oil

   0.5 g of bismuth subgallate will displace (1 × 0.5) ÷ 2.5 g of theobroma oil = 0.2 g

Therefore, the weight of base required to make medicated suppositories = 20 g − 0.2 g = 19.8 g

6   Total weight of the suppositories = 5 × 4 g × 1.2 = 24 g
Weight of hydrocortisone acetate required = (24 g × 1) ÷ 100
= 0.24 g
Therefore, the weight of the base required = 24 g − 0.24 g
= 23.76 g

7   Total weight of morphine hydrochloride required = 8 × 20 mg
= 120 mg = 0.16 g
Weight of base required for unmedicated suppositories = 8 × 2 g
× 1.2 = 19.2 g
As the displacement value of morphine hydrochloride = 1.6,
1.6 g of morphine hydrate displaces 1 g of theobroma oil,
1 g of morphine hydrate displaces 1 ÷ 1.6 g of theobroma oil
and 0.16 g of morphine hydrate displaces (1 × 0.16) ÷ 1.6 g
theobroma oil = 0.1 g of theobroma oil
This means that the drug will displace 0.1 g × 1.2 of the glycerol-
gelatin base = 0.12 g
Therefore, the weight of base required to make medicated
suppositories = 19.2 g − 0.12 g = 19.08 g

8   Total weight of phenobarbitone sodium required = 10 × 30 mg
= 300 mg = 0.3 g
Total weight of unmedicated suppositories = 10 × 1 g × 1.2 = 12 g
As the displacement value of phenobarbitone sodium = 1.2,
1.2 g of phenobarbitone sodium will displace 1 g of theobroma oil
1 g of phenobarbitone sodium will displace 1 ÷ 1.2 g of theobroma
oil, and 0.3 g of phenobarbitone sodium will displace (1 × 0.3) ÷
1.2 g of theobroma oil = 0.25 g of theobroma oil
This means that the drug will displace 0.25 g × 1.2 of the glycerol-
gelatin base = 0.3 g
Therefore, the weight of base required to make medicated
suppositories = 12 g − 0.3 g = 11.7 g

9 Total weight of diphenhydramine hydrochloride required = 12 × 50 mg
= 600 mg = 0.6 g

Total weight of unmedicated suppositories = 12 × 2 g × 1.2
= 28.8 g

As the displacement value of diphenhydramine hydrochloride = 1.2,

1.2 g of diphenhydramine hydrochloride will displace 1 g of theobroma oil

1 g of diphenhydramine hydrochloride will displace 1 ÷ 1.2 g of theobroma oil

0.6 g of diphenhydramine hydrochloride will displace (1 × 0.6) ÷ 1.2 g of theobroma oil = 0.5 g

This means that the drug will displace 0.5 g × 1.2 of glycerol-gelatin base = 0.6 g

Therefore the weight of base required to make medicated suppositories = 28.8 g − 0.6 g = 28.2 g

10 Total weight of bismuth subgallate required = 10 × 50 mg = 500 mg
= 0.5 g

Total weight of hydrocortisone acetate required = 10 × 10 mg
= 100 mg = 0.1 g

Total weight of unmedicated suppositories = 10 × 2 g = 20 g

As the displacement value of bismuth subgallate = 2.5,

2.5g of bismuth subgallate will displace 1 g of theobroma oil

1 g of bismuth subgallate will displace 1 ÷ 2.5 g of theobroma oil

0.5 g of bismuth subgallate will displace (1 × 0.5) ÷ 2.5 g of theobroma oil = 0.2 g of theobroma oil

As the displacement value of hydrocortisone acetate = 1.5,

1.5 g of hydrocortisone acetate will displace 1 g of theobroma oil

1 g of hydrocortisone acetate will displace 1 ÷ 1.5 g of theobroma oil

0.1 g of hydrocortisone acetate will displace (1 × 0.1) ÷ 1.5 g of theobroma oil = 0.06 g of theobroma oil

Total weight of theobroma oil displaced = 0.25 g + 0.06 g = 0.31 g

Therefore, the weight of base required to make medicated suppositories = 20 g − 0.31 g = 19.69 g

Answers to the summary test

1. 0.25 L =   250 mL
 75 mL =   75 mL
 4000 µl =   4 mL
 Total volume = 329 mL

2. Daily, the patient must take 5 mL × 4 = 20 mL
In seven days the patient will take 20 mL × 7 = 140 mL

3. 1 mol of potassium chloride weighs 80 g
Therefore 1 mmol of potassium chloride weighs 80 mg
So, 40 mmol of potassium chloride weighs 40 × 80 mg = 3200 mg
 or 3.2 g

4. 100 g of the cream contains 2 g of salicylic acid
1 g of the cream contains 2/100 g of salicylic acid
350 g of the cream contains 2 × 350/100 g of salicylic acid = 7 g of
 salicylic acid

5. 1 g of adrenaline is dissolved in 10,000 mL of the solution
1 mg of adrenaline is dissolved in 10 mL of the solution
 (10,000/1000)
20 mg of adrenaline is dissolved in 200 mL of the solution

6. 1 g of antiseptic is dissolved in 1000 mL of the mouthwash
1/1000 g of antiseptic is dissolved in 1 mL of the mouthwash
50/1000 g of antiseptic is dissolved in 50 mL of the mouthwash
 = 0.05 g
Daily, the patient uses 0.05 g × 4 of the antiseptic = 0.2 g
In seven days, the patient uses 0.2 g × 7 of the antiseptic = 1.4 g

7 Chloral Elixir Paediatric BP:

Chloral hydrate	200 mg	20 g
Water	0.1 mL	10 mL
Blackcurrant syrup	1 mL	100 mL
Syrup	to 5 mL	to 500 mL

8 Coal Tar and Zinc Ointment BP:

Strong coal tar solution	100 g	15 g
Zinc oxide	300 g	45 g
Yellow soft paraffin	600 g	90 g
Total weight	1000 g	150 g

9 Zinc and Salicylic Acid Paste BP:

Zinc oxide	24%	96 g
Salicylic acid	2%	8 g
Starch	24%	96 g
White soft paraffin	50%	200 g
Total weight	400 g	

10 For the 1:10,000 solution:

1 g of potassium permanganate is dissolved in 10,000 mL of the solution

0.01 g of potassium permanganate is dissolved in 100 mL of the solution

Therefore, the patient is using a 0.01% w/v solution of potassium permanganate

Daily, the patient uses 20 mL × 2 = 40 mL

In 10 days the patient uses 40 mL × 10 = 400 mL

Now apply the dilution formula $C_1 \times V_1 = C_2 \times V_2$:

C_1 = 4% w/v

V_1 = ?

C_2 is a 1:10,000 solution of potassium permanganate = 0.01% w/v

V_2 = 400 mL

$4 \times V_1 = 0.01 \times 400$

$4 \times V_1 = 4$

$V_1 = 1$ mL

11 Use $C_1 \times M_1 = C_2 \times M_2$:

$C_1 = 2\%$ w/w

$M_1 = 400$g

$C_2 = 0.5\%$ w/w

$M_2 = ?$

$2 \times 400 = 0.5 \times M_2$

Therefore, $M_2 = 1600$ g

Hence, in order to carry out the dilution, we must add $1600 - 400 = 1200$ g of emulsifying ointment

12 $\dfrac{\text{Initial weight of drug} + \text{added weight of drug}}{\text{Initial volume of solution} + \text{added volume of solution}} = \dfrac{4}{100}$

$\dfrac{0 + x}{500 + \frac{100x}{40}} = \dfrac{4}{100}$

$2000 + 10x = 100x$

$2000 = 90x$

$200 = 9x$

$x = 22.2$ g

22.2 g of dextrose are dissolved in $(100 \times 22.2) \div 40$ mL of the 40% w/v solution = 55.5 mL

13 $\dfrac{\text{Initial weight of drug} + \text{added weight of drug}}{\text{Initial weight of cream} + \text{added weight of drug}} = \dfrac{5}{100}$

Initial weight of drug = 2 g (since we have 200 g of a 1% w/w cream)

Added weight of drug = x g

Initial weight of cream = 200 g

$\dfrac{2 + x}{200 + x} = \dfrac{5}{100}$

$2000 + 10x = 200 + 100x$

$1800 = 90x$

$x = 20$ g

14 First, determine the concentration per millilitre of the bumetanide in the glucose 5% w/v solution. 5 mg in 500 mL = 5000 mcg in 500 mL = 10 mcg/mL. If the maximum rate is 100 mcg/min and 100 mcg can be found in 10 mL of solution, the maximum rate will be 10 mL/min.

15 Determine the amount of dopamine administered over 1 h. If there is 160 mg/50 mL in the original solution and the infusion rate is 5 mL/h, the patient is receiving 16 mg/h. They are therefore receiving 16 mg/h, which is 0.257 mg/min = 267 mcg/min. If the patient weighs 80 kg, they are receiving 267/80 mcg/kg/min = 3.3 mcg/kg/min.

16 First, calculate the patient's ideal body weight (IBW):

IBW (female) = $0.9H - 92 = (0.9 \times 170\text{ cm}) - 92 = 61$ kg

Therefore ABW is lower.

The equation for calculating renal function is:

$$\text{C1}_{cr}\text{ (females)} = \frac{1.04(140 - \text{Age}) \times \text{Weight (kg)}}{\text{Serum creatinine (μmol/L)}}\text{ mL/min}$$

$$= \frac{1.04(140 - 80) \times 60}{170\text{ μmol/L}}\text{ mL/min}$$

$$= 22.2\text{ mL/min}$$

We can therefore assume that this patient has mild renal impairment.

17 Determine the patient's ideal body weight (IBW):

Males IBW = $(0.9 \times H) - 88 = 74$ kg

Therefore the IBW is lower than the ABW.

From Chapter 7, bioavailability of digoxin $F = 0.7$, salt fraction $S = 1$ and volume of distribution per kilogram of lean body weight is $V_d/\text{kg} = 7.3$ L/kg

From the question the target concentration C is 2.1 mcg/1

Loading dose $= \frac{C \times V_d}{F \times S}$

$$\frac{1.2\text{ mg/L} \times 7.3\text{ L/kg} \times 74\text{ kg}}{0.7 \times 1} = 1620.6\text{ mcg}$$

Hence 1500 mcg digoxin tablets could be prescribed.

18 From the last question, the patient's IBW was calculated to be 74 kg. We know from Chapter 7 that $F = 0.7$ for digoxin tablets, $S = 1$, from the question the target concentration $C = 1.2$ mcg/L, renal function $Cl_{cr} = 18$ mL/min and dosage internal $\tau = 24$ h. First, determine the digoxin clearance for a patient with congestive heart failure. From Chapter 7:

$$\text{Digoxin clearance (mL/min)} = 0.33 \times \text{Weight (kg)} + 0.9\, Cl_{cr}$$
$$= (0.33 \times 74\text{ kg}) + (0.9 \times 18\text{ mL/min})$$
$$= 40.6\text{ mL/min}$$
$$= 2.4\text{ L/h}$$

Finally, calculate the recommended maintenance dose:

$$\text{Maintenance dose} = \frac{\text{Digoxin clearance (L/h)} \times \text{Concentration (mcg/1)} \times \tau}{\text{Bioavailability } (F) \times \text{Salt fraction } (S)}$$

$$= \frac{2.4\text{ L/h} \times 1.2\text{ mcg/1} \times 24\text{ h}}{0.7 \times 1}$$

$$= 172.8\text{ mcg daily}$$

187.5 mcg could be prescribed on a daily basis.

19 Weight of bismuth subgallate required $= 12 \times 100$ mg $= 1.2$ g
Weight of base required for unmedicated suppositories $= 12 \times 4$ g
   $= 48$ g
As the displacement value of bismuth subgallate $= 2.4$,
2.4 g of bismuth subgallate will displace 1 g of theobroma oil,
1 g of bismuth subgallate will displace $1 \div 2.4$ g of theobroma oil,
1.2 g of bismuth subgallate will displace $(1 \times 1.2) \div 2.4$ g of
   theobroma oil $= 0.5$ g
Therefore, weight of base required to make medicated suppositories
   $= 48$ g $- 0.5$ g $= 47.5$ g

20 Total weight of the suppositories $= 10 \times 2$ g $\times 1.2 = 14$ g
Weight of hydrocortisone acetate required $= (14$ g $\times 0.5) \div 100 =$
   0.07 g
Therefore, weight of the base required $= 14$ g $- 0.07$ g $= 14.93$ g